Hot Topics in Acute Care Surgery and Trauma

Series Editors

Federico Coccolini
General, Emergency and Trauma Surgery Department
Pisa University Hospital
Pisa, Italy

Raul Coimbra
Riverside University Health System Medical Center
Riverside, USA

Andrew W. Kirkpatrick
Department of Surgery and Critical Care Medicine
Foothills Medical Centre
Calgary, AB, Canada

Salomone Di Saverio
Department of Surgery (Addenbrooke)
Cambridge University Hospitals NHS Foundation Trust
Cambridge, Cambridgeshire, UK

Editorial Board

This series covers the most debated issues in acute care and trauma surgery, from perioperative management to organizational and health policy issues.

Since 2011, the founder members of the World Society of Emergency Surgery's (WSES) Acute Care and Trauma Surgeons group, who endorse the series, realized the need to provide more educational tools for young surgeons in training and for general physicians and other specialists new to this discipline: WSES is currently developing a systematic scientific and educational program founded on evidence-based medicine and objective experience. Covering the complex management of acute trauma and non-trauma surgical patients, this series makes a significant contribution to this program and is a valuable resource for both trainees and practitioners in acute care surgery.

More information about this series at http://www.springer.com/series/15718

Michael Sugrue • Ron Maier
Ernest E. Moore • Fausto Catena
Federico Coccolini • Yoram Kluger
Editors

Resources for Optimal Care of Emergency Surgery

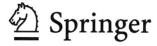
Springer

Editors
Michael Sugrue
General Surgery Department
Letterkenny University Hospital
Letterkenny
Donegal
Ireland

Ernest E. Moore
Ernest E Moore Shock Trauma Center
Denver Health
Denver, CO
USA

Federico Coccolini
General, Emergency and Trauma Surgery
Department
Pisa University Hospital
Pisa
Italy

Ron Maier
Department of Surgery
Harborview Medical Center
Seattle, WA
USA

Fausto Catena
Emergency and Trauma Surgery
Ospedale di Parma
Parma
Italy

Yoram Kluger
Department of General Surgery
Rambam Health Care Campus
Haifa
Israel

ISSN 2520-8284   ISSN 2520-8292   (electronic)
Hot Topics in Acute Care Surgery and Trauma
ISBN 978-3-030-49365-3   ISBN 978-3-030-49363-9   (eBook)
https://doi.org/10.1007/978-3-030-49363-9

This Springer imprint is published by the registered company Springer Nature Switzerland AG
The registered company address is: Gewerbestrasse 11, 6330 Cham, Switzerland

Foreword

Research is fundamentally altering the daily practice of acute care surgery (trauma, surgical critical care, and emergency general surgery) for the betterment of patients around the world. Management for many diseases and conditions is radically different than it was just a few years ago. For this reason, concise up-to-date information is required to inform busy clinicians. Therefore, since 2011 the World Society of Emergency Surgery (WSES), in partnership with the American Association for the Surgery of Trauma (AAST), endorses the development and publication of the "Hot Topics in Acute Care Surgery and Trauma", realizing the need to provide more educational tools for young in-training surgeons and for general physicians and other surgical specialists. These new forthcoming titles have been selected and prepared with this philosophy in mind. The books will cover the basics of pathophysiology and clinical management, framed with the reference that recent advances in the science of resuscitation, surgery, and critical care medicine have the potential to profoundly alter the epidemiology and subsequent outcomes of severe surgical illnesses and trauma.

Federico Coccolini
General, Emergency and Trauma Surgery Department
Pisa University Hospital
Pisa, Italy

Raul Coimbra
Riverside University Health System – Med
Riverside, CA, USA

Andrew W. Kirkpatrick
Department of Surgery and Critical Care Medic
Foothills Medical Centre
Calgary, AB, Canada

Salomone Di Saverio
Department of Surgery (Addenbrooke)
Cambridge University Hospitals NHS Foundation Trust
Cambridge, UK

Preface

Emergency surgery care delivery is a cornerstone of medicine, enshrined in a culture of curing patients presenting to our hospitals with a wide variety of emergency conditions. Managing acute admissions and presentations to emergency rooms, optimally from the outset, in a timely fashion with appropriate resources offers the best chance for cure.

Surgery and its increasingly interdisciplinary team approach to the emergency patient offers that hope. This books engenders a process of suggesting benchmarks and performance indicators to stimulate improvements in care processes and outcomes. Engagement with health administrators, governments and most importantly with the community is vital in moving forward. Emergency general surgery conditions take many lives. It accounts for over 10% of all hospital admissions and has evolved to medicine's "poor cousin", falling behind the advances and leadership in other medical fields, particular trauma and injury. The chapters in this book provide some leadership to move forward.

Our patients need us to advocate for change, where possible evidence based, giving them the best chance of survival with minimal morbidity and at a reasonable cost.

Letterkenny, Donegal, Ireland	Michael Sugrue
Seattle, WA, USA	Ron Maier
Denver, CO, USA	Ernest E. Moore
Parma, Italy	Fausto Catena
Pisa, Italy	Federico Coccolini
Haifa, Israel	Yoram Kluger

The original version of the book was revised: Affiliation of one of the editors, Ernest E. Moore, has been updated. The correction to the book is available at https://doi.org/10.1007/978-3-030-49363-9_26

Contents

Part I Key Position Topics

**1 Position Paper on Designation of Resources for Emergency
   Surgery Services** 3
   Li Hsee, George Velmahos, Philip Crowley, and Ken Mealy

2 Acute Care Surgery Unit Structure 9
   Federico Coccolini, Ron Maier, Ernest E. Moore, Luca Ansaloni,
   Timothy Hodgetts, and Paul Balfe

3 Optimal Care in Geriatric Emergency Surgery (GES) 15
   Mihai Paduraru

4 Sepsis: Control and Treatment 23
   Massimo Sartelli

5 Resuscitation in Emergency General Surgery 29
   Liam S. O'Driscoll, Alison Johnston, Noel Hemmings,
   Michael Sugrue, and Manu L. N. G. Malbrain

6 Medical Laboratory Support for Emergency Surgery 51
   Maurice O'Kane

7 Radiology and Emergency Surgery 55
   Gavin Sugrue, Ruth M. Conroy, and Michael Sugrue

**8 Interaction Between Gastroenterology and Emergency General
   Surgery** 61
   Chris Steele, Paula Loughlin, Angus Watson, and Michael Sugrue

**9 Advanced and Specialist Nursing Practice in Emergency
   Surgery: The Team Approach** 63
   Randal Parlour, Carol-Ann Walker, Louise Flanagan,
   and Paula Loughlin

**10 Data, Registry, Quality Improvement and Patient Outcome
   Measures** 71
   Sam Huddart

11   **Research in Emergency General Surgery**........................ 83
     Fausto Catena, Gennaro Perrone, Elena Bonati,
     Antonio Tarasconi, Andrew Kirkpatrick, and Ron Maier

12   **Position Paper on Education and Training in Emergency
     Surgery**... 89
     Michael Sugrue, Mark W. Bowyer, Leo Lawler,
     Isidro Martinez, and Lyndsay Pearce

13   **Appendicitis**.. 95
     Gaetano Poillucci, Mauro Podda, Stavros Gourgiotis,
     and Salomone Di Saverio

14   **Acute Mesenteric Ischemia** 103
     Miklosh Bala and Jeffry Kashuk

15   **Intra-abdominal Hypertension and Abdominal Compartment
     Syndrome: Updates**... 115
     Bruno M. Pereira and Pablo R. Ottolino-Lavarte

Part II   Key Performance Indicators

16   **Cholecystitis**.. 131
     Luca Ansaloni, Louise Flanagan, and Michael Sugrue

17   **Pancreatitis** 133
     Ari Leppaniemi

18   **Upper GI Bleed** 137
     Chris Steele

19   **Bowel Obstruction** 139
     Randal Parlour, Manvydas Varzgalis, and Brendan Skelly

20   **Perforated Gastroduodenal Ulcer (PGDU)** 141
     Kjetil Soreide

21   **Acute Diverticulitis (AD): Management Phase** 145
     Marja Boermeester

22   **Abdominal Vascular Emergencies**.............................. 149
     Scott Thomas

23   **Coagulation** 153
     Ernest E. Moore

24   **Wound Care**.. 155
     Michael Sugrue

25   **Complications in Emergency Surgery**.......................... 157
     Michael Sugrue, Kevin Blake, Brendan Skelly,
     and Angus J. M. Watson

Correction to: Resources for Optimal Care of Emergency Surgery C1

Part I

Key Position Topics

Position Paper on Designation of Resources for Emergency Surgery Services

Li Hsee, George Velmahos, Philip Crowley, and Ken Mealy

1.1 Introduction

Timely access to emergency surgery presents a major health challenge worldwide. Patients requiring emergent and urgent surgical care are often critical. Some cases are life-threatening, therefore prompt attention is required. Due to the wide spectrum of surgical conditions, timely input from clinicians with the right expertise, a multi-disciplinary approach and a streamlined acute pathway are critical to ensure optimal outcomes for patients.

Historically, it is not uncommon to manage emergency surgical patients interspersed in the daily elective activities within a given hospital system [1]. The lack of timely access to emergency surgical care is a growing problem. The reasons for this are often multi-factorial and may include shortage of emergency surgeons, inadequate access to operating room and lack of a dedicated team and clinical pathway [2].

L. Hsee (✉)
Auckland City Hospital, Auckland, New Zealand
e-mail: LiH@adhb.govt.nz

G. Velmahos
Massachusetts General Hospital, Boston, MA, USA
e-mail: GVELMAHOS@mgh.harvard.edu

P. Crowley
Quality Improvement, Dr Steevens' Hospital, Dublin, Ireland
e-mail: philip.crowley@hse.ie

K. Mealy
Wexford General Hospital, Wexford, Ireland

Royal College of Surgeons in Ireland, Dublin, Ireland

National Clinical Programme in Surgery, Dublin, Ireland
e-mail: kmealy@rcsi.ie

© World Society of Emergency Surgery and Donegal Clinical and Research Academy 2020   3
M. Sugrue et al. (eds.), *Resources for Optimal Care of Emergency Surgery*,
Hot Topics in Acute Care Surgery and Trauma,
https://doi.org/10.1007/978-3-030-49363-9_1

Over the past decade, the importance of a comprehensive system in managing emergency surgical care is better recognised across the health sector and government organisations. Surgical colleges, hospital institutions, training boards and health ministries have published multiple consensus papers and statements on this topic.

The aim of this paper is to outline the minimum requirement of resources and designation on emergency surgery services. This aim is also to identify important key performance indicators to facilitate the validation of emergency surgical care in order to provide a safe delivery of surgical care for acute patients.

1.2   Methods

A review of published articles and consensus statements relating to the establishment and design of emergency, acute care surgery and emergency general services was performed. Emergency surgery position statements from the surgical colleges, surgical institutions and key government organisations were assessed. Key elements of the emergency resource allocation and designation were identified. Five key performance indicators were developed according to the standardisation of this position paper.

1.3   Results

The emerging organisation of an emergency surgery service as a distinct entity is advocated and supported by surgical colleges and health organisations. The overarching aim is to improve and streamline overall acute patient care and maximise patient outcomes.

The development and configuration of an emergency surgical service should not be implemented in isolation [3]. While there is no set format or structure of an acute surgical delivery, the following is an outline of a framework, which summarises the principles of the resources and designation of emergency surgery:

1.3.1   Identify the Scope of Emergency Surgical Requirements

There is evidence that the quality of emergency patient care is varied and suboptimal worldwide [4]. Contributing factors include lack of infrastructure, resources, senior clinical input, leadership and management. The emergency surgical workload is often high and under-appreciated. In order to provide adequate resources for an emergency surgical service, it is important to understand the scope of service requirement such as patient volume, case mix and level of clinical support. Surgical demand and access need to be measured routinely [5]. This can be achieved through training, research and planning of health services [6]. The workload of emergency surgery can then be predicted and measured.

1.3.2   Leadership

Clinical leadership in emergency surgery is paramount and needs to be identified early on. The appointment should be an experienced surgeon who has a clear understanding of the acute surgical process and a commitment to quality surgical care. Clinical governance is achieved through the support and partnership of surgical colleagues, senior hospital management and often the institutional chief executive [7]. An appointed steering group may be beneficial to advocate for the resources of an emergency surgical service.

1.3.3   Patient Care

There should be a balance between elective and emergency surgical streams. Patient-centred care often requires a separation of emergency surgical patient care from elective settings [8]. Emergency surgical resources need to be protected and ring-fenced to that effect. A clear acute surgical pathway from admission to discharge must be recognised and developed [9]. Timely access to investigations, diagnostic and pathology services contribute to the efficiency of an emergency service [10]. Where possible a dedicated operating room and sessions must be made available to the emergency surgical service. Emergency surgical care is led by consultant surgeons to provide timely and accurate decision-making and treatment [7]. There is a potential to decrease health care costs by reducing unnecessary investigations [11]. Emergency surgical cases, where clinically appropriate, should be scheduled during standard hours. The aim is to reduce unnecessary surgery after hours and overnight [6]. There is evidence that prolonged hours increases the risk of serious errors that can lead to patient harm and death [6]. A multi-disciplinary approach to the overall care of the patient is vital. This would include nurse specialist and allied health providers.

1.3.4   Emergency Surgical Team and Supporting Staff

While there is no set team structure, emergency surgical team design depends on the cohort of patients, case mix and resources available. Appropriately trained and competent health care professionals are required to provide the service. The consultant surgeon should not have other commitments while managing the emergency surgical service [6]. It is ideal for surgical trainees to gain competency in the management of emergency surgical patients. It is also valuable to involve nursing colleagues. A multi-disciplinary radiology meeting dedicated to emergency surgical service will provide education and improve patient care [1]. Sufficient administrative support must be employed to facilitate the team.

1.3.5 Training

While the aim is to improve surgical patient care, there is an opportunity to provide training of emergency surgeons. This allows surgical fellows and senior residents to obtain concentrated expertise in the acute and emergency aspects of surgery. As emergency surgical service is a consultant led service, it facilitates the supervision of residents, interns and medical students. It is also an invaluable field for training in surgical nursing and emergency anaesthesiology. Accreditation is required in emergency surgical training. Many surgical colleges have already incorporated emergency surgical training into their curriculum [12]. Studies have shown that certified emergency programmes improve outcomes in patients undergoing emergency surgery.

1.3.6 Patient Follow-Up, Benchmarking and Quality Initiatives

Follow-up for patients post discharge from the emergency surgical service is an integral part of emergency surgical care. Monitoring includes factors such as histology, wound reviews and further patient assessments. Participation in departmental mortality and morbidity audits is essential. Data collection and interval reviews of key performance indicators are also valuable [13]. Surgical services should benchmark common measures for service and patient care improvement.

1.3.7 Designation of Emergency Surgical Services

An increasing number of tertiary care hospitals are utilising a dedicated emergency surgical service with sub-specialty support. In urban and rural settings, regionalisation of acute care has been supported. Its aim is to provide not only the best care of the patients in the specialty but also support for outlying community hospitals where complex surgical conditions can be transferred [14]. It is a safety net for the improvement of emergency surgical patient care. While regionalisation and designation policies are complex with multiple competing issues, careful planning and evaluations are required [15]. A localised policy and regional escalation plan is necessary to facilitate communication and resource utilisation [16].

1.4 Conclusion

This position paper outlines the minimum standards and principles of framework required for resources and designation of emergency surgical services. The provision of emergency surgical care is constantly evolving. Existing policies and resources require constant evaluation to ensure the optimal care of the emergency surgical patient.

References

1. Hsee L, Devaud M, Middleberg L, Jones W, Civil I. Acute Surgical Unit at Auckland City Hospital: a descriptive analysis. ANZ J Surg. 2012;82(9):588–91.
2. Association of Surgeons of Great Britain and Ireland. Emergency general surgery: the future a consensus statement [Internet]. ASGBI. 2007. http://www.asgbi.org.uk/en/publications/consensus_statements.cfm
3. Royal Australasian College of Surgeons. The case for the separation of elective and emergency surgery [Internet]. RACS. 2011. http://www.surgeons.org/media/college-advocacy/. Accessed 29 Mar 2016.
4. Santry HP, Madore JC, Collins CE, Ayturk MD, Velmahos GC, Britt LD, et al. Variations in implementation of acute care surgery: results from a national survey of university-affiliated hospitals. J Trauma Acute Care Surg. 2015;78(1):60–7.
5. Charles J, Jones A. Key messages from the literature [Internet]. Public Health Wales. 2012. http://www.wales.nhs.uk/sitesplus/836/documentmap/. Accessed 29 Mar 2016.
6. Department of Health, State Government of Victoria. A framework for emergency surgery in victorian public health services [Internet]. Victoria State Government. 2012. https://www2.health.vic.gov.au/about/publications/policiesandguidelines/A%20framework%20for%20emergency%20surgery%20in%20Victorian%20public%20health%20services. Accessed 29 Mar 2016.
7. Sorelli PG, El-Masry NS, Dawson PM, Theodorou NA. The dedicated emergency surgeon: towards consultant-based acute surgical admissions. Ann R Coll Surg Engl. 2008;90:104–8.
8. The Royal College of Surgeons of England. Separating emergency and elective surgical care: recommendations for practice [Internet]. RCSENG professional standards and regulation. 2007. http://www.rcseng.ac.uk/publications/docs/separating_emergency_and_elective.html. Accessed 29 Mar 2016.
9. Hameed SM, Brenneman FD, Ball CG, Pagliarello J, Razek T, Parry N, et al. General surgery 2.0: the emergence of acute care surgery in Canada. Can J Surg. 2010;53(2):79–83.
10. Professional Standards and Regulation Directorate: Royal College of Surgeons of England. Standards for unscheduled surgical care: guidance for providers, commissioners and service planners [Internet]. Publications Department, The Royal College of Surgeons of England. 2011. https://www.rcseng.ac.uk/publications/docs/emergency-surgery-standards-for-unscheduled-care. Accessed 29 Mar 2016.
11. Gale SC, Shafi S, Dombrovskiy VY, Arumugam D, Crystal JS. The public health burden of emergency general surgery in the United States: a 10-year analysis of the nationwide inpatient sample—2001 to 2010. J Trauma Acute Care Surg. 2014;77(2):202–8.
12. Pearce L, Smith SR, Parkin E, Hall C, Kennedy J, Macdonald A. Emergency general surgery: evolution of a subspecialty by stealth. World J Emerg Surg. 2016;11:2.
13. Royal College of Surgeons in Ireland. Model of care for acute surgery: national clinical programme in surgery [Internet]. RCSI. 2013. https://www.rcsi.ie/ncps-acutesurgery. Accessed 29 Mar 2016.
14. Diaz JJ, Norris PR, Gunter OL, Collier BR, Riordan WP, Morris JA. Does regionalization of acute care surgery decrease mortality? J Trauma. 2011;71(2):442–6.
15. Block EF, Rudloff B, Noon C, Behn B. Regionalization of surgical services in central Florida: the next step in acute care surgery. J Trauma. 2010;69(3):640–3. Discussion 643–4.
16. Santry HP, Janjua S, Chang Y, Petrovick L, Velmahos GC. Interhospital transfers of acute care surgery patients: should care for nontraumatic surgical emergencies be regionalized? World J Surg. 2011;35(12):2660–7.

Acute Care Surgery Unit Structure

2

Federico Coccolini, Ron Maier, Ernest E. Moore,
Luca Ansaloni, Timothy Hodgetts, and Paul Balfe

Acute care surgery (ACS) refers to the surgical management of emergency conditions, requiring some form of immediate surgical care or intervention. Essentially ACS should offer the surgeon the opportunity to acquire a working diagnosis, to intervene appropriately and thereby to promptly have an impact on the outcome of the critically ill patient [1]. The last decade has seen a major advance in the field of ACS in most developed countries, and to some extent this has become the standard of care worldwide. The evolution of ACS units in order to effectively manage patients presenting with acute surgical emergencies presents an enormous challenge not only to the medical profession, but also to all healthcare providers and medical institutions, as well as placing an immense strain on the National

The original version of the book was revised: Affiliation of one of the editors, Ernest E. Moore, has been updated. The correction to the book is available at https://doi.org/10.1007/978-3-030-49363-9_26

F. Coccolini (✉)
General, Emergency and Trauma Surgery Department, Pisa University Hospital, Pisa, Italy

R. Maier
Harborview Medical Center, Seattle, WA, USA
e-mail: ronmaier@uw.edu

E. E. Moore
Ernest E Moore Shock Trauma Center, Denver Health, Denver, CO, USA
e-mail: Ernest.Moore@dhha.org

L. Ansaloni
Unit of General and Emergency Surgery, Bufalini Hospital of Cesena, AUSL Romagna, Cesena, Forlì-Cesena, Italy

T. Hodgetts
HQ Allied Rapid Reaction Corps, Army Role 1 Champion, Innsworth, Gloucester, UK
e-mail: timothy.hodgetts793@mod.gov.uk

P. Balfe
St. Luke's Hospital, Kilkenny, Ireland

© World Society of Emergency Surgery and Donegal Clinical and Research Academy 2020   9
M. Sugrue et al. (eds.), *Resources for Optimal Care of Emergency Surgery*,
Hot Topics in Acute Care Surgery and Trauma,
https://doi.org/10.1007/978-3-030-49363-9_2

Healthcare Systems. It should always be emphasized that at the center of these issues is the patient [1–4]. In many hospitals of different countries, surgical emergencies are still managed by an on-call team, which is also responsible for elective surgery.

Regrettably in this model, surgical emergencies are often attended to after the elective commitments have been completed. This is obviously far from ideal, thus opening a new pathway for ACS to develop and improve. Historically there have been several factors which have contributed to the development of ACS as a separate entity:

1. First, over the last 20 years there has been a progressive trend for general surgeons to subspecialize, i.e., general surgeons have wanted to focus their interest on a particular area in general surgery, such as gastrointestinal surgery, vascular surgery, or bariatric surgery. Most of this work is in the form of elective surgery. As a result, surgeons have become de-skilled in managing patients with acute surgical emergencies.
2. Second, there was an established urgent need to improve the quality of care given to patients with surgical emergencies. Traditionally surgical emergencies were managed by a team of doctors who were on-call for that day or week for emergencies, but who also had elective commitments in the form of an elective theatre list or an outpatient clinic. As a result the emergencies were only attended to after the elective commitments had been attended to. This invariably resulted in considerable delays in the management of the emergencies and it almost invariably occurred after normal working hours. The overall impact was that these patients with surgical emergencies often received suboptimal care.
3. Third, there is a trend for older surgeons to not want to do emergency calls and to operate in the middle of the night. As a result, it has become increasingly difficult to maintain an adequate roster of general surgeons on-call for emergencies.
4. Finally, the impact of the increasing conservative approach to many trauma conditions has decreased the operative experience of trauma surgeons. For example, many patients with blunt abdominal trauma can now be managed non-operatively. As a result, the amount of surgery being performed by trauma surgeons has decreased considerably and trauma surgeons are becoming de-skilled.

For these reasons, Acute Care Surgery Units (ACSU) should be developed in order to provide acute surgical management in a timely manner, i.e., management which includes both diagnostic and therapeutic services. Cases include emergency abdominal surgery, such as removal of the gallbladder or appendix, management of acute bowel obstruction, and reduction of, and surgical intervention for acute hernias. It often incorporates the surgical management of life-threatening infections.

Several different ACS models for providing care for surgical emergencies have been described:

1. Combination of acute surgical care, trauma, and critical care: In this case, ACS has been described as a multidisciplinary approach involving Emergency and Trauma Surgery, and Critical Care Medicine [5–7]. This model would be ideally applicable in a setting where the trauma load is small or to hospitals which do not have a stand-alone trauma unit.
2. Dedicated, stand-alone ACS (non-trauma): This model would apply to institutions that have a dedicated stand-alone trauma unit, carrying a substantive trauma load.
3. Team of dedicated on-call doctors (1 week at a time), where the team would be free of their normal elective commitments for that week: This model would be applicable to most hospitals.

When considering a global view, the development of an ACS model has been driven mostly by research and literature from the USA and some European countries. The USA and Europe have diverse opinions and ideas on the various issues related to ACS, with the two parts always analyzing developments on either side of the Atlantic. One of the clear differences is the terms of employment and compensation of doctors, which determines the extent to which emergency call is mandatory or voluntary. The USA relies on the basic emergency service that is provided by residents and interns, compared to being covered by fully trained consultant. This permits the latter to concentrate more on elective surgery, but also offers the residents more chances to practice skills and techniques. The European system differs in that doctors are generally employed directly by hospitals and must take calls on the basis of a duty roster, thus covering all fields of emergency and elective surgery [8–10].

In most hospitals in the USA, surgical emergencies include trauma and acute surgical diseases, as well as incorporating critical care as part of their functional unit. This ACS paradigm is estimated to relieve some of the stress on the surgical staff, aiming at maintaining or improving patient care and increasing the attractiveness of trauma and emergency surgery to surgical trainees [11]. The mixture of emergency and general surgical care by trauma units has allowed the trauma surgeon to maintain operative skills in an era of increased non-operative management [12].

The various models of ACS are well recognized in the literature. At the one end of the range is Ernest E Moore Shock Trauma Center at Denver Health in Denver, Colorado, where the work of the acute, trauma, and critical care are combined as a single service [13]. At the other end are institutions which have separate services for trauma, emergency surgery, and critical care. Between these two extremes are institutions which base their service on the number of surgeons existing and the variety of surgical disease presenting at the institution. These institutions may have a two- or more-team approach to the treatment of their patient populations, often combining their trauma and emergency surgery services, at the same time maintaining a separate critical care service [14, 15]. In response to the need for better access to urgent surgical care and other pressing issues, such as the workforce shortage, one of the potential solutions could be the creation of ACS as a subspecialty, even in the model of organization [16]. Even from the educational point of view, as treatment paradigms shift to ACS and emergency surgical disease management evolves, there will be a need for properly trained surgeons, who are willing to pursue the optimal urgent care (surgical or conservative) for these conditions. In addition to this, as the amount of knowledge available in medical science has grown exponentially, it has become increasingly difficult to be an expert in every aspect of general surgery after only 4 or 5 years of training. This has contributed to the current fragmentation manifesting as a plethora of subspecialty disciplines [6, 17, 18]. ACSU should contribute to create a surgeon able to afford the efficacious care for all surgical emergency conditions.

The initial driving force behind the specialty in trauma care was the special need for the injured patient. Thus the special needs of the severely ill surgical patient, requiring emergency intervention, should be used as the driving force in recognizing the need for the ACSU. Regardless of how ACS is administered, the aim is that the trauma or non-trauma related acute surgical patient receives optimal care from the moment of presentation until discharge [4, 11].

In consequence of these premises, the "ideal" structure of an ACSU can be described as a modular structure. The modular units dedicated with a 24 h provision which essentially make up an ACSU are the following:

1. A modular units for emergency acceptance of patients with emergency resuscitation resources (i.e., shock trauma room).
2. A modular unit for emergency diagnostics (ultrasounds, traditional radiology, CT scan…).
3. Theatre and other interventional resources (e.g., interventional angiography).
4. ICU (for intensive management during observation, conservative treatment and postoperative period).
5. Non-intensive surgical modular unit (for non-intensive management during observation, conservative treatment and postoperative period).

Depending on locally available resources, these modular units can be variously reassembled, but essentially they must at least have a shared protocol of coordination (Fig. 2.1).

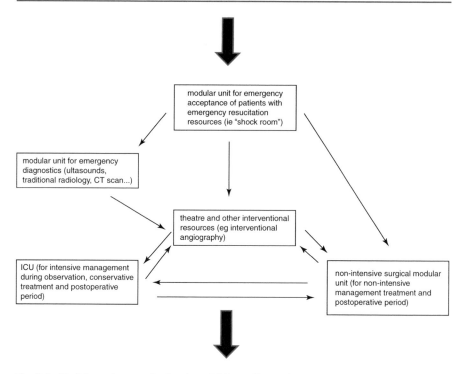

Fig. 2.1 Modular units organizational model (according to local resources, these modular units can be variously reassembled)

References

1. Earley AS, et al. An acute care surgery model improves outcomes in patients with appendicitis. Ann Surg. 2006;244:498–504.
2. Trunkey DD. In search of solutions. J Trauma. 2002;53:1189–91.
3. Buckley J. The shame of emergency care for kids. US News World Rep. 1992;112:34–43.
4. Rontondo MF. At the center of the—perfect storm II: the patient. Surgery. 2007;141:291–2.
5. Schwab CW. Crises and war: stepping stones to the future. J Trauma. 2007;62:1–16.
6. Søreide K, Nedrebø BS. Recruitment problems in the surgical specialty? Tidsskr Nor Laegeforen. 2008;128(16):1852–3.
7. Borman KR, et al. Changing demographics of residents choosing fellowships: longterm data from the American Board of Surgery. J Am Coll Surg. 2008;206:782–8. discussion, 788–9
8. Catena F, Moore E. WSES and the role of emergency surgery in the world. World J Emerg Surg. 2007;2:3.
9. De Waele JJ, Hoste EA. The future of surgical critical care: a European perspective. Crit Care Med. 2007;35:984–6.
10. Pascual J, et al. American College of Surgeons criteria for surgeon presence at initial trauma resuscitations: superfluous or necessary? Ann Emerg Med. 2007;50:15–7.

11. Uranues S, Lamont E. Acute care surgery: the European model. World J Surg. 2008;32:1605–12.
12. Spain DA, et al. Should trauma surgeons do general surgery? J Trauma. 2000;48:433–8.
13. Moore EE. Acute care surgery: the safety net hospital model. Surgery. 2007;141:297–8.
14. Austin MT, et al. Creating an emergency general surgery service enhances the productivity of trauma surgeons, general surgeons and the hospital. J Trauma. 2005;58:906–10.
15. Davis KA, et al. Trauma team oversight of patient management improves efficiency of care and augments clinical and economic outcomes. J Trauma. 2008;65:1236–44.
16. Representatives of the participating organizations in Congress. Acute care congress on the future of emergency surgical care in the United States. J Trauma. 2009;67:1–7.
17. Davis KA, Rozycki GS. Acute care surgery in evolution. Crit Care Med. 2010;38(9 Suppl):S405–10.
18. Søreide K. Trauma and the acute care surgery model—should it embrace or replace general surgery? Scand J Trauma Resusc Emerg Med. 2009;17:4.

Optimal Care in Geriatric Emergency Surgery (GES)

3

Mihai Paduraru

3.1 Putting Things in Context

Population ageing—the increasing share of older persons in the population—is one of the most significant social transformations of the twenty-first century. Globally, the number of older persons is growing faster than the number of people in any other age group and this has important implications for nearly all sectors of society, especially in developed countries [1].

3.1.1 What Do We Mean by 'Elderly'?

This is an arbitrary numerical definition which is subject to a number of variables. In developing countries, the chronological age of 50+ is used as a definition of elderly by the World Health Organization; however, for developed countries, 65+ years is more acceptable [2]. From the surgical point of view, 'biological age' also has to be taken substantially into consideration since the combined effects of genetics, social and/or physical environment and chronological age impact on the physiological reserve of an individual. Gerontologists have recognized the very different conditions that people experience as they grow older and sub-grouping the 'elderly' into 'young-old' (65–74), 'middle-old' (75–84), and 'oldest-old' (85+) can be beneficial in helping to accommodate need more specifically.

M. Paduraru (✉)
Milton Keynes University Hospital NHS Foundation Trust,
Milton Keynes, Buckinghamshire, UK
e-mail: Mihai.Paduraru@mkuh.nhs.uk

© World Society of Emergency Surgery and Donegal Clinical and Research Academy 2020   15
M. Sugrue et al. (eds.), *Resources for Optimal Care of Emergency Surgery*,
Hot Topics in Acute Care Surgery and Trauma,
https://doi.org/10.1007/978-3-030-49363-9_3

3.1.2 Demographical Perspective

The most recent study undertaken by the United Nations reports that, by 2030, one in six people (16.5%) worldwide will be aged 60 years or over and that by 2050 this ratio will increase to one in five. In 2015, it was one in eight and it is clear to see that the pace of world population ageing is accelerating. Significantly, in Europe, older persons are expected to account for more than 25% of the population by the year 2030 [1].

A slightly different focus given by the European Commission calculates that *the demographic old-age dependency ratio* (people aged 65 or above relative to those aged 15–64) has risen from 25% in 2010 to 29.6% in 2016 and is projected to eventually reach 51.2% in 2070 [3].

Globally, the number of people aged 80 years or over is growing even faster than the number of older persons overall. Projections indicate that in 2050 this age group will have more than tripled in number since 2015 and will account for more than 20% of the global population and in Europe, this number is expected to reach 23% by 2030 [1]. In the EU, life expectancy at birth for males is expected to increase from 78.3 (2016) to 86.1 by 2070 and in females from 83.7 to 90.3 [3].

3.2   What is the Problem?

It is indisputable that as the number and proportion of elderly people within the population increases, the demand on healthcare will be exponentially greater with a significant impact on emergency geriatric surgery. The hypothesis that morbidity rather than mortality will increase due to projected longer life expectancy creates a real challenge for health services. The elderly are living for longer with their co-morbidities, which increases the surgical risk, hospital length of stay and the cost of care.

3.2.1   Profile of the Elderly Patient

As the age of the patient increases, they are more likely to present as emergency rather than elective cases and with a range of pre-existing medical conditions. Up to 74% of elderly emergency surgical patients have been found to have two or more chronic medical conditions, strongly associated with increased age and frailty [4]. The National Confidential Enquiry into Patient Outcome and Death found that for patients over the age of 80 who died within 30 days of admission, 31.2% of cases had abdominal surgery and 83.4% of cases were admitted as an emergency, rather than electively [5]. This is due in the main to a certain degree of reluctance to perform elective surgery earlier in older (and poly-morbid) patients considered to be high risk.

It has to be acknowledged however that the acute abdomen in the elderly patient is challenging to diagnose. This is partly due to the typical features one would expect in certain intra-abdominal conditions not presenting themselves and the patient having reduced or atypical pain or absence of signs in intra-abdominal sepsis [6]. Other important contributing factors are communication impediments—auditory and ability to express symptoms—and delayed referral to the hospital due to limited mobility and dependency. Such 'delays' inevitably result in a deterioration of the patient's condition, an increase in risk factors and a need now for emergency surgery (ES), with little to no option of whether to operate or not at this stage.

3.2.2 Emergency Laparotomy

Emergency laparotomy is a common procedure with more than 30,000 being performed annually in the UK. High-risk patients are classified as those with a $\geq 5\%$ risk of mortality, which equates to around two-thirds of patients [7]. Half of the operations performed are in the elderly and in 2012 carried a mortality of 20% at 30 days, six times more than in those patients under 50 and 24.4% in patients aged 80 or over [8].

3.2.3 Main Emergency Surgical Pathologies in Elderly Patients

- Diverticulitis becomes more common with age and presents in more than 60% of patients over 80; with high post-operative morbidity and mortality when surgery is required.
- Biliary disease can be difficult to diagnosis with delays leading to complications including empyema, gallbladder perforation and severe biliary sepsis. The mortality rate of elderly patients diagnosed with cholecystitis is approximately 10%.
- Small bowel obstruction on adhesions is common in those elderly having previous operations. Sigmoid volvulus is also common in immobile aged patients. Risk factors include chronic constipation, institutionalization, antipsychotic and other constipating medication.
- Colorectal is one of the three most common cancers in elderly males and females and is more likely to be presented as an emergency, mostly as obstructive tumours.
- Acute mesenteric ischemia typically presents later in life. Intestinal necrosis (acidosis, hypotension and high lactate) can develop and be fatal.
- Vascular emergencies: AAA is most common in 70+ and 80+ year olds; it has a 75% mortality rate with age being an independent risk factor [6].

3.2.4 Medical Associated Illness

In GES, the often common complex dual problem of the surgical pathology and medical co-morbidity (mainly cardiovascular and respiratory chronic disease) opens the door to surgical and medical post-operative complications.

This interaction between medical and surgical is often based on a reciprocal aggravating mechanism, increasing the complexity to one greater than the sum of its parts and leaving geriatric emergency surgery with the highest surgical mortality rates.

Co-morbidities coupled with a degree of cognitive impairment, poly-pharmacy, poor nutrition and restricted mobility all contribute to increased patient frailty, which is an independent predictor of post-operative morbidity and mortality more specific than the chronological age alone [9]. It has been assessed that as high as 37% of the elderly emergency surgical population are classed as frail [10] and 70% of older acute surgical patients have cognitive impairment [11].

3.2.5 Post-operative Complications

'The patient may tolerate an operation, but not a complication' is a well-known aphorism. One of the main post-surgical morbidities in GES is ileus with a higher risk of vomiting and, consequently, aspiration. This increases the risk for post-operative pneumonia and sepsis with fatal consequences in many cases.

A further post-operative complication, specifically in the elderly and interrelated with the above, is post-operative delirium. This is characterized by a disturbance of consciousness and a change in cognition that develop over a short period of time and has also been associated with restricted mobility, pressure ulcers and pulmonary emboli. In addition, it appears to be an important marker for risk of dementia (or death), even in older people without prior cognitive or functional impairment [9].

3.3   How Do We Improve?

The need to improve emergency surgery outcomes and by implication GES, has been highlighted through several national reports and guidance documents from lead bodies in the UK in the last two decades [7, 12–14]. These include hospital management with adequate staffing, and support; and ES as a separate, specialist area with its own dedicated surgeons with full 24 h, 7 days a week consistently high and accessible levels of service. These aspects *general* to emergency surgery, once addressed, will solve part of the problem and have a positive effect on GES outcomes.

Measures to improve emergency surgery outcomes in recent years have started to be implemented. NELA (National Emergency Laparotomy Audit) measures delivery of care based on multidisciplinary standards. They monitor identification of risk of death before surgery; timely consultant reviews of the patient with surgery performed under the direct care of a consultant surgeon; and prompt and ready access to investigations and essential support services, treatment and theatres (24 h availability) [7].

However, due to the fact that the higher morbid-mortality in elderly emergency surgical patients is multi-factorial, part of the problem *specific* to GES, a multi-modal approach is needed to improve it. Elderly emergency patients need to be treated as a specific subgroup, requiring a specifically tailored and proactive approach.

This approach can be summarized into four main areas: preoperative; surgical decision making; post-operative; and infrastructure and staffing.

A word about ERAS

Enhanced Recovery after Surgery programmes, evidenced-based protocols, are designed to standardize and optimize perioperative care in order to reduce surgical complications, perioperative physiological stress and organ dysfunction (metabolic, endocrine and inflammatory response as well as reduce protein catabolism). There is substantial evidence in the literature demonstrating the effectiveness of these measures in elective surgery to reduce morbidity and mortality in elderly patients [15]. Based on this, the RCS recommends the implementation of ERAS in GES [14] and there is some evidence in relation to ERAS in ES generally [16] and with older (>70) patients more specifically, to show that it is feasible and safe for these patients and results in fewer post-operative complications [17]. However, ERAS needs to be modified in ES.

3.3.1 Preoperative

Here the focus is on identifying patient risk through assessment and ideally, undertaking pre-habilitation in order to optimize the patient for surgery. The Royal College of Surgeons (RCS) recommends comprehensive geriatric assessment (CGA) undertaken by multi-disciplinary teams (MDTs) for elderly patients [14] and NELA recommends that all patients aged over 70 years should undergo an assessment of multi-morbidity, frailty and cognition—associated with frailty and post-operative delirium—to guide further input from MDTs [7].

In preoperative GES, one important challenge is time management. Preoperative optimization might need to include correcting clotting, effective hemodynamic stabilization and assessment/adjustment of long-standing medication as priorities.

Any assessment clearly needs to be as efficient as possible. P-Possum is frequently used in the emergency laparotomy setting as an effective predictor of post-operative mortality. Frailty assessment, including cognitive impairment, as a key element in CGA, along with P-Possum, could be an effective and expedient method for predicting risk [18]. There are a number of modified and quick to administer tests available which are reported to be effective in predicting degrees of frailty and mortality in acute, elderly patients.

It is important to stress that risk assessment tools should be used to help guide but not be the only criterion on which the decision to operate or not is based. In the end, even when the patient's risk score is very high, surgery may still be the only life-saving option.

3.3.2 Surgical Decision Making

Although age or multi-morbidity is not a barrier to surgical intervention [4], the decision-making process in elderly emergency surgical patients (especially in the frail) should be guided by a minimum aggressiveness and maximum effectiveness approach.

Interventional and conservative management approaches need to be considered more in order to avoid ES mortality in elderly patients. These should include gall-bladder drainage in severe cholecystitis (Tokyo Guidelines 2018) and stenting in obstructive bowel cancers.

3.3.3 Post-operative Rehabilitation

Reducing the use of sedatives and major tranquillizers and opioids, avoiding routine post-operative drainage and implementing early oral feeding, as well as helping the patient to be mobilized as quickly as possible, are appropriate and implementable measures, with the aid of dedicated, specialized staff, in the post-operative rehabilitation of GES patients.

All these measures have also been linked to reducing post-operative delirium and are recommended measures by geriatric specialists [19].

3.3.4 Staff and Infrastructure

The importance of senior clinical staff involvement in high-risk patients as well as smooth team working between accident and emergency departments, surgeons, anaesthetists, theatres, critical care units and wards is indisputable. For GES (and ES), the early and direct involvement of the consultant is essential. Furthermore, hospitals need to provide facilities and allocated staffing to proactively encourage early post-operative mobilization of the patient.

Finally, it has already been highlighted that there is a need for specifically dedicated and specially trained staff at all levels and these might be best placed in distinct units or specialist centres and headed by a specialist consultant.

Positive examples of the benefit of specialist centres and units can be found in the Geriatric Centre at The Mount Sinai Hospital and the Multidisciplinary Unit for the Surgical Management of Geriatric Patient in Barcelona, Spain [20].

3.4 Conclusions

GES is a 'new old problem'; the issues and how to manage it have attained critical status as the effects of the impact of the demographic shift are being felt. The response to this problem has to be dynamic. ES has to have 'sub-specialty status' and GES has to be an area of interest within it, with distinct measures, resources and practice, in order to deliver optimum care.

References

1. United Nations, Department of Economic and Social Affairs, Population Division. World population ageing. 2015 (ST/ESA/SER.A/390).
2. Proposed working definition of an older person in Africa for the MDS project. http://www.who.int/healthinfo/survey/ageingdefnolder/en/
3. The 2018 ageing report: underlying assumptions and projection methodologies. European Commission Directorate-General for Economic and Financial Affairs.
4. Hewitt J, McCormack C, Tay HS, et al. Prevalence of multimorbidity and its association with outcomes in older emergency general surgical patients: an observational study. BMJ Open. 2016;6:e010126.
5. National Confidential Enquiry into Patient Outcome and Death (NCEPOD). An age old problem: a review of the care received by elderly patients undergoing surgery. 2010.
6. Torrance ADW, Powell SL, Griffiths EA. Emergency surgery in the elderly: challenges and solutions. Open Access Emerg Med. 2015;7:55–68.
7. NELA Project Team. Third patient report of the National Emergency Laparotomy Audit RCoA London. 2017.
8. Saunders DI, Murray D, Pichel AC, Varley S, Peden CJ. Variations in mortality after emergency laparotomy: the first report of the UK Emergency Laparotomy Network. Br J Anaesth (England). 2012;109:368–75.
9. Moug SJ, Stechman M, McCarthy K, Pearce L, Myint PK, Hewitt J. Frailty and cognitive impairment: unique challenges in the older emergency surgical patient. Ann R Coll Surg Engl. 2016;98(3):165–9.
10. Joseph B, Zangbar B, Pandit V, Fain M, Mohler MJ, Kulvatunyou N, et al. Emergency general surgery in the elderly: too old or too frail? J Am Coll Surg. 2016;222(5):805–13.
11. Hewitt J, Williams M, Pearce L, et al. The prevalence of cognitive impairment in emergency general surgery. Int J Surg. 2014;12:1031–5.
12. Nuffield Trust (Commissioned by Royal College of Surgeons). Emergency general surgery: challenges and opportunities. 2016.
13. Association of coloproctology of GB and Ireland/Association of UGI surgeons and association of surgeons of GB and Ireland. The future of emergency general surgery: a joint document. 2015.
14. The Royal College of Surgeons. Emergency surgery policy briefing. 2014.
15. Bagnall NM, Malietzis G, Kennedy RH, Athanasiou T, Faiz O, Darzi A. A systematic review of enhanced recovery care after colorectal surgery in elderly patients. Color Dis. 2014;16:947–56.
16. Paduraru M, Ponchietti L, Casas IM, Svenningsen P, Zago M. Enhanced recovery after emergency surgery: a systematic review. Bull Emerg Trauma. 2017;5(2):70–8.
17. Paduraru M, Ponchietti L, Casas IM, Svenningsen P, Pereira J, Landaluce-Olavarria A, et al. Enhanced recovery after surgery (ERAS)—the evidence in geriatric emergency surgery: a systematic review. Chirurgia (Bucur). 2017;112(5):546–57.
18. Sharrock AE, McLachlan J, Chambers R, Bailey IS, Kirkby-Bott J. Emergency abdominal surgery in the elderly: can we predict mortality? World J Surg. 2017;41:402–9. https://doi.org/10.1007/s00268-016-3751-3.
19. American Geriatrics Society. Clinical practice guideline for postoperative delirium in older adults. J Am Geriatr Soc. 2015;63(1):142–50.
20. Parés D, Fernandez-Llamazares J. Unidades funcionales para el manejo quirurgico del paciente geriá trico. Cir Esp. 2018;96:129–30.

Sepsis: Control and Treatment

4

Massimo Sartelli

4.1 Introduction

Sepsis is a complex, multifactorial syndrome which can evolve into conditions of varying severity. If left untreated, it may lead to the functional impairment of one or more vital organs or systems. Therefore its adequate treatment is crucial already in the emergency room.

Early detection and timely therapeutic intervention can improve the overall clinical outcome of septic patients; reducing time to diagnosis of sepsis is thought to be a critical component in reducing mortality from multiple organ failure. However, early diagnosis of sepsis can be difficult; determining which patients presenting with signs of infection during an initial evaluation do currently have, or will later develop, a more serious illness is challenging.

Despite decades of sepsis research, no specific therapies for sepsis have emerged. Without specific therapies, management is based on control of the infection and organ support. Fluid resuscitation and support of vital organ function, early antibiotics, and source control are the cornerstones for the treatment of patients with sepsis.

In February 2016, the Journal of the American Medical Association (JAMA) published a proposal for new definitions and criteria for sepsis, called Sepsis-3 [1], updating previous sepsis definitions.

Sepsis is now defined as life-threatening organ dysfunction caused by a dysregulated host response to infection. It can be clinically represented by an increase in the Sequential Organ Failure Assessment (SOFA) score of 2 points or more [1].

Septic shock is defined as a subset of sepsis in which particularly profound circulatory, cellular, and metabolic abnormalities are associated with a greater risk of mortality than with sepsis alone. Patients with septic shock can be clinically identified by a vasopressor requirement to maintain a mean arterial pressure of 65 mmHg

M. Sartelli (✉)
Department of Surgery, Macerata Hospital, Macerata, Italy

© World Society of Emergency Surgery and Donegal Clinical and Research Academy 2020   23
M. Sugrue et al. (eds.), *Resources for Optimal Care of Emergency Surgery*,
Hot Topics in Acute Care Surgery and Trauma,
https://doi.org/10.1007/978-3-030-49363-9_4

or greater and serum lactate level greater than 2 mmol/L (>18 mg/dL) in the absence of hypovolemia [1].

Under this terminology, "severe sepsis" becomes superfluous.

Furthermore, the consensus group proposed the introduction of qSOFA as an alert system. Patients with at least 2 of 3 clinical abnormalities including Glasgow coma score of 14 or less, systolic blood pressure of 100 mmHg or less, and respiratory rate 22/min or greater may be prone to have the poor outcome typical of sepsis. Importantly, qSOFA does not define sepsis but provides simple bedside criteria to screen adult patients with suspected infection.

Sepsis should generally warrant greater levels of monitoring and intervention.

In patients with severe sepsis or septic shock, the Surviving Sepsis Campaign (SSC) guidelines recommend [2]: (1) that treatment and resuscitation begin immediately, (2) that administration of IV antimicrobials be initiated as soon as possible after recognition and within 1 h for both sepsis and septic shock, and (3) that a specific anatomic diagnosis of infection requiring emergent source control be identified or excluded as rapidly as possible in patients with sepsis or septic shock.

4.2 Hemodynamic Resuscitation

It is well known that early treatment with aggressive hemodynamic support can limit the damage of sepsis-induced tissue hypoxia and prevent the overstimulation of endothelial activity.

Early, adequate hemodynamic support of patients in shock is crucial to prevent worsening organ dysfunction and failure.

Fluid therapy to improve microvascular blood flow and increase cardiac output is an essential part of the treatment of sepsis.

A fluid challenge incorporates four determinant elements [3]:

1. Crystalloid solutions should be the first choice, because they are well tolerated and cheap.
2. Fluids should be infused rapidly to induce a quick response but not so fast that an artificial stress response develops.
3. The goal should be an increase in systemic arterial pressure.
4. Pulmonary edema is the most serious complication of fluid infusion and appropriate monitoring is necessary to prevent its occurrence.

Vasopressor agents should be administered to restore organ perfusion if fluid resuscitation fails to optimize blood flow in various organs.

It may be acceptable practice to administer a vasopressor temporarily while fluid resuscitation is ongoing, with the aim of discontinuing it, if possible, after hypovolemia has been corrected although the benefit of this approach is unclear [3].

Norepinephrine is now the first-line vasopressor agent used to correct hypotension in the event of septic shock [2]. It is more efficacious than dopamine and is more effective for reversing hypotension in patients with septic shock [2]. Moreover, dopamine may cause tachycardia more frequently and may be more arrhythmogenic than norepinephrine.

Dobutamine is another inotropic agent that increases cardiac output, regardless of whether norepinephrine is also being given. With predominantly β-adrenergic properties, dobutamine is less likely to induce tachycardia than either dopamine or isoproterenol [3].

Hypotension is the most common indicator of inadequate perfusion and restoring a mean arterial pressure of 65–70 mmHg is a good initial goal during the hemodynamic support of patients with sepsis [3].

Hemodynamic resuscitation has been the cornerstone of management for severe sepsis and septic shock in Surviving Sepsis Campaign guidelines since its first draft [4].

Rivers et al. [5] demonstrated that early goal-directed therapy (EGDT), initiated in the emergency department, reduced the in-hospital mortality rates of patients in septic shock. However, results of recent multi-center prospective randomized trials [6–8] have been unable to reproduce the Rivers' results [9].

EGDT involved reaching a target ScvO2 ≥ 70% (through transfusion of red cells and dobutamine). Patients should otherwise have: central venous pressure (CVP) ≥8–12 mmHg (through crystalloid boluses), mean arterial pressure (MAP) ≥65 mmHg (through vasopressor administration), urine output ≥0.5 mL/kg/h (whenever possible). Early identification of sepsis and prompt administration of intravenous fluids and vasopressors are always mandatory. However, initial resuscitation should not be based on a simple, predetermined protocol.

Restoring a mean systemic arterial pressure of 65–70 mmHg is a good initial goal during the hemodynamic support of patients with sepsis.

4.3   Antimicrobial Therapy

A key component of the initial management of the septic patient is the administration of IV empiric antimicrobial therapy. An insufficient or otherwise inadequate antimicrobial regimen is strongly associated with unfavorable outcomes in critically ill patients [10].

Empiric broad-spectrum antimicrobial therapy should be started as soon as possible in all patients with sepsis or septic shock. In these patients, dosing strategies of antimicrobials should be always optimized based on accepted pharmacokinetic/pharmacodynamic principles and specific drug properties [2].

Accurate diagnostic tests are essential for the correct identification of microorganisms causing sepsis.

The performance of antimicrobial susceptibility testing by the clinical microbiology laboratory is crucial both to confirm susceptibility to the empirical therapy, and to detect resistance in bacterial isolates. At least two sets of blood cultures for both aerobic and anaerobic bacteria and fungal organisms should always be obtained before starting empirical antimicrobial therapy.

4.4   Source Control

Source control encompasses all measures undertaken to eliminate the source of infection, reduce the bacterial inoculum, and correct or control anatomic derangements to restore normal physiologic function [11, 12].

Patients with sepsis need to be carefully examined to ensure that all drainable foci have been identified. Infected fluid collections, devitalized tissue, and devices may act as a persistent source of sepsis until removed.

It is well known that inadequate source control at the time of the initial operation has been associated with increased mortality in patients with severe intra-abdominal infections [13].

4.5   Conclusion

Sepsis is a complex condition that is often life-threatening. Early recognition of sepsis and early intervention are paramount in improving outcomes.

A systematic, organized approach to identify and control sepsis is mandatory to improve the outcomes of patients.

References

1. Singer M, Deutschman CS, Seymour CW, Shankar-Hari M, Annane D, Bauer M, et al. The third international consensus definitions for sepsis and septic shock (sepsis-3). JAMA. 2016;315(8):801–10.
2. Rhodes A, Evans LE, Alhazzani W, Levy MM, Antonelli M, Ferrer R, et al. Surviving sepsis campaign: international guidelines for management of sepsis and septic shock: 2016. Intensive Care Med. 2017;43(3):304–77.
3. Vincent JL, De Backer D. Circulatory shock. N Engl J Med. 2013;369(18):1726–34.
4. Dellinger RP, Carlet JM, Masur H, et al. Surviving sepsis campaign guidelines for management of severe sepsis and septic shock. Crit Care Med. 2004;32:858–73. [Errata, Crit Care Med. 2004;32:1449, 2169–70].
5. Rivers E, Nguyen B, Havstad S, et al. Early goal-directed therapy in the treatment of severe sepsis and septic shock. N Engl J Med. 2001;345:1368–77.
6. ProCESS Investigators, Yealy DM, Kellum JA, Huang DT, Barnato AE, Weissfeld LA, et al. A randomized trial of protocol-based care for early septic shock. N Engl J Med. 2014;370(18):1683–93.
7. Mouncey PR, Osborn TM, Power GS, Harrison DA, Sadique MZ, Grieve RD, et al. Trial of early, goal-directed resuscitation for septic shock. N Engl J Med. 2015;372(14):1301–11.
8. ARISE Investigators, ANZICS Clinical Trials Group, Peake SL, Delaney A, Bailey M, Bellomo R, et al. Goal-directed resuscitation for patients with early septic shock. N Engl J Med. 2014;371(16):1496–506.
9. De Backer D, Vincent JL. Early goal-directed therapy: do we have a definitive answer? Intensive Care Med. 2016;42(6):1048–50.
10. Sartelli M, Catena F, Di Saverio S, Ansaloni L, Malangoni M, Moore EE, et al. Current concept of abdominal sepsis: WSES position paper. World J Emerg Surg. 2014;9(1):22.
11. Marshall JC. Principles of source control in the early management of sepsis. Curr Infect Dis Rep. 2010;12(5):345–53.

12. Marshall JC, al Naqbi A. Principles of source control in the management of sepsis. Crit Care Clin. 2009;25(4):753–68.
13. Sartelli M, Chichom-Mefire A, Labricciosa FM, Hardcastle T, Abu-Zidan FM, Adesunkanmi AK, et al. The management of intra-abdominal infections from a global perspective: 2017 WSES guidelines for management of intra-abdominal infections. World J Emerg Surg. 2017;12:29.

Resuscitation in Emergency General Surgery

5

Liam S. O'Driscoll, Alison Johnston, Noel Hemmings, Michael Sugrue, and Manu L. N. G. Malbrain

5.1 Introduction

Patients who require emergency general surgery often present with shock, which may be further compounded by the presence of comorbidities. In elective surgery, pre-operative assessment allows optimisation of comorbidities and improvement in functional status to reduce morbidity and mortality associated with surgery and anaesthesia. For patients requiring emergency general surgery, timely recognition and treatment of shock is crucial to reduce the morbidity and mortality associated to the shock state as well as the stress of emergency surgery.

L. S. O'Driscoll (✉)
Department of Anaesthesia, Letterkenny University Hospital,
Letterkenny, Co. Donegal, Ireland

A. Johnston
Donegal Clinical Research Academy, Letterkenny University Hospital,
Letterkenny, Co. Donegal, Ireland

EU INTERREG Emergency Surgery Outcomes Advancement Project (eSOAP),
Letterkenny University Hospital, Letterkenny, Co. Donegal, Ireland
e-mail: Alison.Johnston@hse.ie

N. Hemmings
Department of Anaesthesia, Altnagelvin Hospital, Derry, UK
e-mail: noel.hemmings@westerntrust.hscni.net

M. Sugrue
Department of Surgery, Emergency Surgery Outcome Advancement Project Centre for
Personalised Medicine, Letterkenny University Hospital and Donegal Clinical Research
Academy, Letterkenny, Donegal, Ireland

Manu L. N. G. Malbrain
Vrije Universiteit Brussel (VUB), Brussels, Belgium

© World Society of Emergency Surgery and Donegal Clinical and Research Academy 2020   29
M. Sugrue et al. (eds.), *Resources for Optimal Care of Emergency Surgery*,
Hot Topics in Acute Care Surgery and Trauma,
https://doi.org/10.1007/978-3-030-49363-9_5

Resuscitation should take place in an appropriately staffed environment, which allows monitoring of the patient, and should occur under the supervision of medical staff familiar with the principles of resuscitation. The ultimate goal of resuscitation is to optimise tissue perfusion with an adequate concentration of oxyhaemoglobin to prevent tissue ischaemia. Management of hypovolaemic, haemorrhagic and septic shock will be described here, with special consideration to the acute general surgical patient.

Coagulopathy is a complication of acute massive haemorrhage as a result of consumption of clotting factors and platelets, haemodilution by resuscitative fluids, and can evolve into disseminated intravascular coagulation (DIC). DIC also complicates sepsis in some patients. The assessment and management of coagulopathy are described.

5.2   Shock States in Emergency Surgical Patients

The US definition states that shock is systolic hypotension <90 mmHg refractory to fluid administration. The European definition defines shock as a mismatch between oxygen delivery and consumption. Shock is a state of cellular and tissue hypoxia due to inadequate oxygen delivery, impaired oxygen diffusion, or increased oxygen utilisation. Shock states arising in emergency surgical patients are varied as a result of the different pathophysiological processes at play in this heterogonous group of patients. For example, in acute small or large bowel obstruction *hypovolaemic shock* is present because of vomiting and sequestration of large volumes of fluid in the bowel lumen. In patients with peritonitis or other infective processes, *distributive shock* may occur as a result of the endothelial dysfunction seen in the overwhelming inflammatory response associated with sepsis and the presence of third space fluid sequestration (ascites). Furthermore, *haemorrhagic shock*, a subset of hypovolaemic shock, is seen in those with acute upper/lower gastrointestinal bleeding or trauma to an abdominal solid organ (spleen, liver), viscus or blood vessel. There may also be combinations of the above described, often associated with translocation of gut bacteria into the circulation as a result of bowel wall distension in bowel obstruction.

Regardless of the pathological process, shock is clinically recognised by the presence of some or all of hypotension (systolic blood pressure < 90 mmHg), tachycardia (>110/min), tachypnoea (>22/min), reduced level of consciousness (GCS <15), oliguria (<0.5 mL/kg/h), hyperlactataemia (>2 mmol/L), reduced capillary refill time (>2 s) and mottling of the skin. Assessing the intravascular volume status of a shocked patient is challenging. In addition, there are many misconceptions, and diagnosis of hypovolaemia is difficult at the bedside. Intravascular versus interstitial hypovolaemia need to be differentiated from one another. Furthermore, hypovolaemia does not always equal dehydration and the presence of fluid responsiveness does not always necessitate fluid resuscitation [1]. These subtleties of volume assessment aside, patients in whom signs of shock are present should be attended to immediately and managed in a high dependency area until transfer to the operating theatre for surgical management of the underlying pathology.

5.3   Principles of Management of the Shocked Patient

Treatment of haemodynamic status should begin while investigation of the underlying cause of shock is ongoing. Early involvement of critical care medicine and anaesthetic teams as part of the surgical response is essential. Oxygen should be administered to increase oxygen delivery and to prevent pulmonary hypertension (related to hypoxic pulmonary vasoconstriction) [2]. Endotracheal intubation and mechanical ventilation are often required in those with dyspnoea, hypoxaemia, or persistent or worsening acidaemia (either metabolic or hypercapnic in origin). Clinicians must be vigilant as cardiovascular collapse can occur in the severely hypovolaemic patient who transitions from negative pressure ventilation to positive pressure ventilation as a result of increased intrathoracic pressure impeding venous return. This is often evidenced by functional haemodynamic monitoring with increased pulse pressure variation (PPV) and stroke volume variation (SVV).

Fluid resuscitation should follow a fluid challenge technique, with haemodynamic and metabolic reassessment of the patient between each fluid bolus (4 mL/kg/10 min) [3]. When approaching resuscitation with intravenous (IV) fluids, it is important to remember that fluids should be seen as any other medication, with indications and contra-indications, and possible adverse effects. A structured conceptual approach should be taken to the use of IV fluids. The 4 D's of fluid therapy (drug–dose–duration–de-escalation) is analogous to the approach taken to antibiotic therapy and is a useful tool. Choice of the drug relates to choice of fluids type: crystalloid versus colloid solutions, isotonic versus hypertonic. Balanced isotonic crystalloid solutions are first choice in resuscitation of hypovolaemic and septic patients (e.g. Ringers lactate or Hartmann's solution). Albumin can be used in hypoalbuminaemic patients. Hydroxyethyl starches are no longer recommended [3, 4]. Five per cent of dextrose also has no role as a resuscitation fluid. Caution must be exercised in the use of 0.9% saline, as infusion of large volumes can cause a hyperchloraemic metabolic acidosis, that is directly related to increased morbidity and worse outcomes [3]. However, in patients who have been vomiting, a hypochloraemic metabolic alkalosis may exist at presentation, and 0.9% saline would be an appropriate choice in this circumstance.

The dose of fluid chosen relates to the particular pharmacokinetics and pharmacodynamics of the chosen fluid, and the current clinical state of the patient. The pharmacokinetics of IV fluids depends on the volume of distribution, osmolality, tonicity, oncoticity and kidney function. For example, if a litre of 5% dextrose, balanced crystalloid, or colloid is administered, at one hour 10%, 25–30%, or 100% of the administered volume remains in the intravascular space, respectively. However, this is influenced by conditions such as inflammation, trauma, blood pressure and infection [3]. Endothelial permeability to colloids is pronounced in sepsis, meaning they offer no benefit over crystalloids [4]. The ratio of colloid to crystalloid to achieve the same haemodynamic response is predicted to be 1:3–1:5. However, trials have shown the observed ratio to be 1:1.3–1:1.5 [5]. The rate of fluid administration also has a bearing on the haemodynamic response to a fluid bolus, and should be such as to induce a measurable response. A rate of 250 mL (4 mL/kg) over

10–15 min or 500 mL over 15–30 min is reasonable. Overly fast rates of infusion can cause endothelial glycocalyx damage resulting in worsening endothelial leak, as well as endothelial shear stress with release of vasoactive substances such as nitric oxide (NO), which result in vasodilation [6].

When one considers the pharmacodynamics of fluid administration, one is describing the relationship between cardiac preload and cardiac output, which in turn requires an understanding of the haemodynamic mechanism of venous return. Most of the circulating blood volume is located in the venous side of the circulation, containing approximately 70% of the body's blood volume. Venous vascular beds consist of unstressed (70%) and stressed (30%) volume. The unstressed volume can be considered as haemodynamically inactive and represents a blood reserve volume (or reservoir). The stressed volume is the remainder of the blood volume in the venous circulation, and the pressure that exists in this stressed volume is known as the mean systemic filling pressure (Pmsf). Venous return is determined by the difference in driving pressure between the Pmsf and the central venous pressure. Thus, when Pmsf is reduced, venous return is reduced, and cardiac output may become impaired when compensatory mechanisms become overwhelmed. The stressed volume can be increased by decreasing vascular capacitance (e.g. by vasopressors), which recruits unstressed volume into stressed volume, and thereby increasing the Pmsf [7]. This is the equivalent of an auto-transfusion (Fig. 5.1).

In the hypovolaemic patient, as the stressed volume increases, either through addition of volume to the system in the form of IV fluids or by decreasing the capacitance of the system through the use of vasopressors to cause venoconstriction, Pmsf is seen to increase resulting ultimately in restored cardiac output. When the total volume of the venous compartment is restored to near euvolaemia, vasopressor requirement may be eliminated. In the patient with septic shock however, vasopressor requirement commonly persists after 30 mL/kg of fluids, making the decision to stop fluid resuscitation more complex and nuanced. Moreover, one size does not fit all and in some patients 30 mL/kg of IV fluid will be too little while it may be too much in others (e.g. those with underlying heart failure) [8].

Duration of fluid therapy should be guided by the ongoing fluid responsiveness of the patient. The definition of fluid responsiveness is a 15% increase in cardiac output after IV fluids. In keeping with the principle that IV fluids should be treated as a drug therapy, the fluid responsiveness of the patient must be assessed prior to conducting a fluid challenge. This can be done with functional haemodynamic parameters (like stroke volume variation (SVV) or pulse pressure variation (PPV)), the passive leg raising test, and the end-expiratory occlusion test [3]. Transthoracic echocardiography (TTE) is a non-invasive investigation, which also gives an indication of the filling status of the patient. It can provide useful information with respect to a number of haemodynamic parameters that can be targeted during resuscitation. All these parameters have their indications and pitfalls.

The objective of resuscitation using fluids is to ultimately restore perfusion of end organs. Clinically, the goal is an increase in cardiac index (but often we can only assess systemic arterial pressure), as well as surrogate markers of end organ perfusion such as increased urine output and decreased capillary refill time. An initial

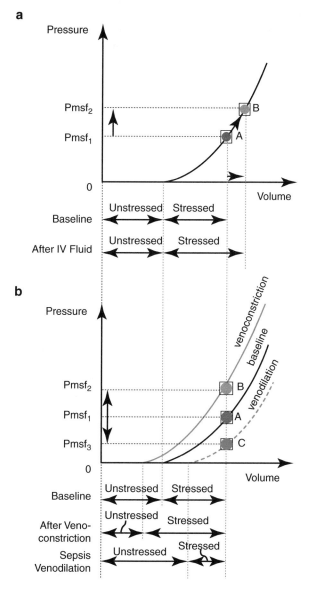

Fig. 5.1 Effect of fluid loading and venoconstriction on volume. (**a**) Effect of volume loading on mean systemic filling pressure (*Pmsf*) and (un)stressed volume. Administration of a fluid bolus increases *Pmsf* (from *Pmsf*1 to *Pmsf*2, indicated respectively by position A (red dot) to B (green dot) on the pressure/volume curve). *Unstressed* volume remains constant while *stressed* volume increases. Total volume = unstressed + stressed increases, carrying a risk for fluid overload. See text for explanation. (**b**) Effect of venoconstriction and venodilation on mean systemic filling pressure (*Pmsf*) and (un)stressed volume. Venoconstriction increases *Pmsf* (from *Pmsf*1 to *Pmsf*2, indicated respectively by position A (red dot) to B (green dot) on the pressure/volume curve). *Unstressed* volume decreases while *stressed* volume increases. Total volume = unstressed + stressed remains constant, resulting in an auto-transfusion effect. Venodilation as seen in sepsis (vasoplegia) decreases *Pmsf* (from *Pmsf*1 to *Pmsf*3, indicated respectively by position A (red dot) to C (blue dot) on the pressure/volume curve). *Unstressed* volume increases while *stressed* volume decreases. Total volume = unstressed + stressed remains constant, resulting in an intravascular underfilling effect. Figure adapted from Jacobs et al. with permission (Open Access CC BY 4.0 licence) [7]

mean arterial pressure (MAP) target of >65 mmHg is usually the goal. However, in patients with chronic arterial hypertension a higher target MAP of 70–80 mmHg may be required to restore adequate tissue perfusion. Reassessment of the status of the patient after each bolus of fluids will help to prevent over-resuscitation, by identifying the appropriate time to de-escalate IV fluid resuscitation. The most important complication of over-resuscitation is acute pulmonary oedema (increased extravascular lung water); however, oedema (and especially venous congestion) can also impair other organ systems including renal function [9]. As the kidney is an encapsulated organ, oedema of the kidney will cause a consequent increased resistance to venous return and contribute to renal ischaemia, with resultant acute kidney injury [10]. Intra-abdominal hypertension leading to abdominal compartment syndrome is also a devastating complication of over-resuscitation with fluids [11, 12]. Vasopressors may be started also while fluid resuscitation is ongoing in order to limit the total amount of fluids administered [2, 4, 13].

5.4 Hypovolaemic Shock

Hypovolaemia arises in the emergency surgical patient as a result of gastrointestinal losses secondary to vomiting and diarrhoea, sequestration of fluid in the bowel lumen in intestinal obstruction, increased insensible losses, increased capillary leak, ascites formation and as a result of haemorrhage. The compensated response to hypovolaemia involves catecholamine-mediated venoconstriction to mobilise reserves from the venous side of the circulation (including the splanchnic circulation), as well as activation of the renin-angiotensin-aldosterone and adrenocorticoid systems to prevent salt and water loss through the urine. Decompensation occurs as volume losses exceed the capacity of these systems to compensate and venous return reduces with an attendant reduction in cardiac output. This manifests clinically as hypotension, and inadequate end organ perfusion (biochemically seen as an increased lactate and decreased base excess).

In hypovolaemia, cardiac output is (normally) preload dependent, on the steep part of the Frank–Starling curve. The goal of fluid resuscitation is not for cardiac output to be preload independent as studies have shown that fluid resuscitation to the point the patient is no longer fluid responsive increases morbidity and mortality [14]. Various tools can be used to assess whether the patient receiving fluid resuscitation continues to be fluid responsive, before the flat part of the Frank–Starling curve has been reached and further fluid resuscitation risks the negative results of over-resuscitation. Insertion of an arterial catheter allows measurement of beat-to-beat arterial blood pressure and pulse pressure variation (PPV). Transthoracic echocardiography can also be used to assess a variety of haemodynamic indices. Insertion of a central venous catheter should also be done to allow measurement of central venous pressure (CVP) and allows sampling of central venous oxygen saturation ($ScvO_2$). However, volumetric preload (e.g. global end-diastolic volume index) may better reflect the true preload status especially in patients with abdominal hypertension.

The PPV is calculated as a percentage difference in the highest and lowest pulse pressures observed on the arterial waveform, and averaged over a couple of respiratory cycles. Many modern patient monitors automatically calculate and display it.

In order to be correctly interpreted, the patient is required to be in a normal sinus rhythm, intubated and mechanically ventilated with tidal volumes of at least 8 mL/kg, making no respiratory effort themselves and in the absence of right heart failure or abdominal hypertension. A PPV value of >12% indicates that the patient is probably fluid responsive (with the present respiratory settings) and in this case an additional fluid bolus may be given when needed (e.g. overt shock or increasing lactate concentration). It is important to ensure that the ventilator settings are correct for the assessment of PPV, and that auto-positive end-expiratory pressure (auto-PEEP) is not present, as this can lead to misinterpretation of the PPV value computed. Another assessment of fluid responsiveness is by performing a passive leg raise. In a hypovolaemic patient, this should result in a transient increase in cardiac output of at least 10% indicating that the patient continues to be fluid responsive.

In mechanically ventilated patients, pulse contour analysis cardiac output monitors can calculate stroke volume (mL), cardiac output (L/min), cardiac index (L/min/m^2), stroke volume variation (%) and systemic vascular resistance (dynes/s/cm^{-5}) continuously (beat-to-beat). These values are derived using the waveform of the arterial pressure (Fig. 5.2). Interpretation of these values may also guide clinical decisions regarding the fluid status and fluid responsiveness of the patient.

As described above, the normal physiological response to hypovolaemia involves activation of the sympathetic nervous system and secretion of endogenous

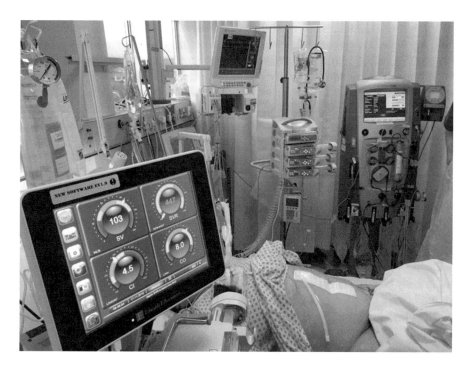

Fig. 5.2 An example of a cardiac output monitor in use in a patient with distributive (septic) shock. Note the signs of hyperdynamic circulatory state—increased stroke volume and cardiac output, with a low systemic vascular resistance (photo credit Michael Sugrue 2019, reproduced with permission)

catecholamines. This results in venoconstriction, recruiting blood from the unstressed volume in the venous side of the circulation. When exogenous vasopressors are infused during resuscitation, their effectiveness is entirely dependent on the remaining blood volume (unstressed volume) in the venous reservoir. Hence, replacing circulating volume should be the priority in the hypovolaemic patient, and vasopressors may only begin to have an effect as circulating volume is increased, as volume is recruited from the unstressed to the stressed volume. However, as resuscitation to near euvolaemia may take hours, it is reasonable to start a vasopressor infusion to achieve a target MAP during ongoing fluid resuscitation, which reduces the duration of hypoperfusion of vital organs.

5.5   Haemorrhagic Shock

Haemorrhagic shock is a subset of hypovolaemic shock and is managed differently. While exsanguination is obvious in external trauma, it may be more difficult to diagnose in those with internal injuries. However, a history of abdominal blunt trauma and hypotension at the time of presentation should raise clinical suspicion of hypovolaemia secondary to bleeding. Uncontrolled bleeding can lead to a systemic consumptive coagulopathy, endothelial damage and haemodilution [15]. The priorities in managing the shocked bleeding patient are mechanical or surgical control of bleeding, monitoring and support of coagulation in a goal-directed treatment strategy, and resuscitation to prevent further tissue ischaemia.

Hypoxaemia should be avoided. Supplemental oxygen should be applied to the awake patient. However, endotracheal intubation may be required as a result of obtundation (GCS <8), hypoxaemia, hypercapnia, or for airway protection. Oxygenation and ventilation targets should be normoxia (SpO_2 > 94%) and normocapnia (5.0–5.5 kPa) on arterial blood gas analysis. Hyperventilation is only indicated in patients with traumatic brain injury in whom transtentorial herniation is imminent [13]. The deadly triad (acidosis, coagulopathy and hypothermia) leading to abdominal hypertension should be avoided at all times [15].

Unlike management of hypovolaemic shock from other causes, haemorrhagic shock management involves permissive hypotension, with a target systolic blood pressure of 80–90 mmHg (MAP 50–60 mmHg) until haemostasis is achieved [15]. A restrictive volume replacement strategy is recommended to achieve the target blood pressure until bleeding is controlled. In addition to fluids, vasopressors may be required to treat life-threatening hypotension to maintain target arterial pressure targets. Isotonic (balanced or buffered) crystalloids are the fluids of choice, and 0.9% saline solutions should be avoided. Colloids (and especially starch solutions) have historically been a mainstay of volume expansion in trauma but their use is no longer recommended due to their adverse effects on haemostasis and kidney function [13].

The target haemoglobin concentration in the acutely bleeding patient is 7–9 g/dL [13]. Initial haemoglobin concentrations may be in the normal range in haemorrhage. Sequestration of interstitial fluid into the vascular compartment takes some time, at which point falling haemoglobin concentrations become evident in laboratory or point-of-care assays. Haemodilution as a result of IV fluid resuscitation also contributes. Tranexamic acid should be given within 3 h after injury in the form of a loading dose of 1 g IV over 10 min followed by 1 g infused over 8 h.

Massive transfusion protocols are varied in the ratios of packed red cells concentrate (RCC), fresh frozen plasma (FFP) and platelets to be given. European guidelines recommend provision of either FFP and RCC in a 1:2 ratio as needed, or fibrinogen concentrate and RCC as needed [13]. However, provision of fixed ratios of blood products in massive haemorrhage is no longer recommended. The advent of point-of-care (POC) prothrombin time tests, rotational thromboelastometry (ROTEM®), thromboelastography (TEG®) and rapid assays of platelet function mean that a more goal-directed strategy may be more prudent where these analysers are available.

ROTEM and TEG are viscoelastic tests of haemostasis allowing measurement of clot formation and dissolution in real time (Fig. 5.3). They provide the same information on clot formation and strength, but use differing terminology to describe

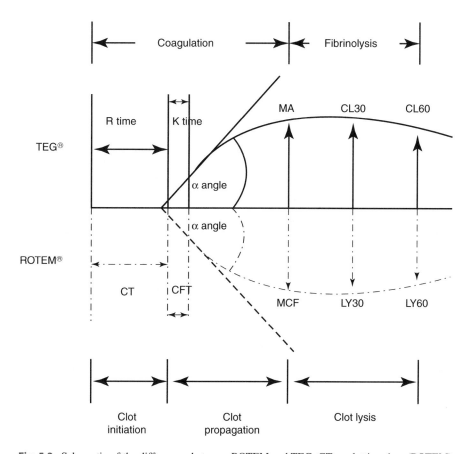

Fig. 5.3 Schematic of the differences between ROTEM and TEG. CT or clotting time (ROTEM) and R (reaction) time (TEG) are the time it takes the clot amplitude to reach 2 mm (first significant clot formation). CFT (clot formation time) and K-time are the time taken for clot amplitude to increase from 2 mm to 20 mm (achievement of a certain clot firmness). The α-angle is a tangent of the initial clot development curve. The maximum clot firmness (MCF) for ROTEM and maximum amplitude (MA) for TEG are the peak amplitudes of the clot (maximum strength of clot). The CL30(60) or LY30(60) indicate the percentage of lysis 30 (respectively 60) min after the MCF/MA. Adapted with permission from Wise et al. [16]

the same parameters. The R-time/CT represents the time to clot initiation and is dependent on clotting factors. The K-time/CFT and α-angles represent properties of clot propagation and are dependent on fibrinogen. The MA/MCF represent the ultimate strength of the clot and is dependent on platelet function as well as fibrinogen.

In variceal and non-variceal upper gastrointestinal bleeding (UGIB), a restrictive transfusion strategy is recommended. A meta-analysis of randomised control trials (RCTs) examining restrictive versus liberal transfusion strategies in all cause UGIB showed higher mortality and rebleeding rates in liberally transfused patients. The restrictive strategies employed a target haemoglobin concentration of 7–8 g/dL. However, in patients with a history of coronary artery disease or recent myocardial ischaemic event, a higher target may be prudent, as the meta-analysis did not adequately examine risk of acute coronary syndrome because it was reported as an outcome measure in only one of the RCTs [17].

5.6 Sepsis and Septic Shock

Sepsis is a medical emergency. It is defined as life-threatening organ dysfunction caused by a dysregulated host response to infection. Septic shock is a subset of sepsis in which underlying circulatory and cellular/metabolic abnormalities are profound enough to increase mortality [18]. The priorities of management of the septic patient are initial resuscitation with IV fluids and vasopressors, early broad-spectrum antibiotics and adequate source control. The Surviving Sepsis Campaign (SSC) have developed care bundles since the publication of the first evidence-based guidelines in 2004. The implementation of such bundles has been shown to reduce mortality [19]. However, blind adherence to the SSC guidelines may induce harm as one size does not fit all [8]. The most recent report in 2018 advocates a "one-hour bundle" which replaces the previous 6-h and 3-h bundles [20]. Table 5.1 outlines the proposed actions that must take place in the first hour after presentation or diagnosis of sepsis. As discussed above, the administration of 30 mL/kg of IV fluids should not be done blindly. Fluids should be given in appropriate boluses (4 mL/kg/10 min) with reassessment of the patient's volume status between boluses.

A patient suspected of having sepsis may require management in a high dependency area prior to transfer to the operating theatre. Critical care physicians should be involved in the early management of this patient group. As hypotension is a prevailing feature of shock, an arterial catheter should be inserted to allow

Table 5.1 The bundle of care to be carried out in the first hour after the diagnosis of sepsis. Reproduced with permission from Levy 2018 [20]

- Measure lactate level. Remeasure if initial lactate is >2 mmol/L.
- Obtain blood cultures prior to administration of antibiotics.
- Administer broad-spectrum antibiotics.
- Begin rapid administration of 30 mL/kg crystalloid for hypotension or lactate ≥4 mmol/L.
- Apply vasopressors if patient is hypotensive during or after fluid resuscitation to maintain MAP ≥65 mmHg.

continuous blood pressure monitoring. It is important to note that vasopressor therapy can be started during fluid resuscitation [2, 4, 13]. Previously it was recommended that vasopressors be started after a patient had failed to have a satisfactory response to 30 mL/kg of IV fluids. The provision of vasopressors at an earlier stage of resuscitation stands to reason—restoration of organ perfusion by whatever means necessary while assessment and fluid resuscitation of the patient is ongoing. While administration of vasopressors via peripheral venous catheters is not best practice, it may be reasonable to start vasopressors peripherally while a central venous catheter is being inserted.

The third international consensus definitions for sepsis and septic shock (Sepsis-3 definitions) have redefined the clinical parameters to aid in the diagnosis of sepsis [18]. Previously, sepsis was defined as the presence of infection or suspected infection with 2 or more systemic inflammatory response syndrome (SIRS) criteria present. The SIRS criteria included presence of two or more of: temperature >38 °C or <36 °C; heart rate > 90/min; respiratory rate > 20/min or $PaCO_2 < 4.3$ kPa; and white blood cell count $>12,000$/mm^3 or < 4000/mm^3 or $>10\%$ immature bands [21]. However, SIRS criteria have poor discriminant and concurrent validity, and the use of the sepsis-related organ failure assessment (SOFA) scoring system provides a more robust set of clinical criteria for the identification of patients with sepsis [18].

The use of the SOFA score was recommended in Sepsis-3, and helps to clinically characterise the septic patient (Table 5.2). It is a proxy for organ dysfunction [22].

Table 5.2 SOFA scoring system. The presence of two points or an increase in two points from baseline identifies those with organ dysfunction as a result of sepsis. Reproduced with permission from Vincent 1996 [22]

SOFA score	1	2	3	4
Respiration				
PaO$_2$/FiO$_2$, mmHg	<400	<300	<200[a]	<100[a]
Coagulation				
Platelets × 10^3/mm^3	<150	<100	<50	<20
Liver				
Bilirubin, mg/dL (μmol/L)	1.2–1.9 (20–32)	2.0–5.9 (33–101)	6.0–11.9 (102–204)	>12.0 (>204)
Cardiovascular				
Hypotension	MAP <70 mmHg	Dopamine ≤5[b] or dobutamine (any dose)	Dopamine >5 or epinephrine ≤0.1 or norepinephrine ≤0.1	Dopamine >15 or epinephrine >0.1 or norepinephrine >0.1
Central nervous system				
Glasgow Coma Scale	13–14	10–12	6–9	<6
Renal				
Creatinine, mg/dL (μmol/L) or urine output	1.2–1.9 (110–170)	2.0–3.4 (171–299)	3.5–4.9 (300–440) or < 500 mL/day	>5.0 (>440) or < 200 mL/day

[a]With ventilatory support
[b]Vasopressor doses are in μg/kg/min

Sepsis is clinically characterised by an acute increase of ≥ 2 SOFA points in the presence of infection. Sepsis-3 also provided clinical criteria for diagnosis of septic shock, which is sepsis with the need for vasopressors to elevate the mean arterial pressure to >65 mmHg and lactate >2 mmol/L despite adequate fluid resuscitation [18]. As the SOFA score requires laboratory results including platelet count, bilirubin and creatinine concentration, and the identification of sepsis requires prompt diagnosis and intervention, the quick-SOFA (qSOFA) score can be used as a screening tool. It incorporates three criteria: altered mentation (GCS <15); systolic blood pressure < 100 mmHg and respiratory rate of ≥ 22/min. A score of 2 or greater helps to identify those patients with infection who require further investigation of organ dysfunction, escalation of therapy, or referral to critical care [18].

5.7 Antibiotics

Current best practice dictates that appropriate antibiotic prophylaxis is administered before the start of surgery [23]. A subset of patients requiring emergency general surgery will have signs of sepsis. Early antibiotics and adequate source control are key determinants of survival in septic shock, with delays in antibiotics being given resulting in increased mortality [24]. The latest guideline from the SSC is that early broad-spectrum antibiotics are given to patients exhibiting signs of sepsis within 1 h of identification of sepsis [20]. For patients who are to undergo emergency general surgery, antibiotics should be given early, rather than waiting for the administration of surgical antibiotic prophylaxis at the start of surgery.

Aerobic and anaerobic blood cultures should be taken before the administration of antibiotics. Sterilisation of blood occurs within minutes of administration of antibiotics [20]. When blood cultures are taken before antibiotic administration, identification of the causative pathogen is more likely, allowing narrowing the spectrum of antibiotics to agents with specific activity against the identified pathogen. This is in keeping with good antimicrobial stewardship principles. In addition to blood cultures, the measurement of pro-calcitonin levels at the time of diagnosis of sepsis may help to reduce duration of antibiotic treatment, and should be part of the initial battery of tests requested (including other biomarkers of infection such as white cell count and C-reactive protein) [25]. Pro-calcitonin is a novel biomarker of bacterial infection. In the resuscitative phase, it may also help to distinguish patients with shock secondary to hypovolaemia from those with shock secondary to sepsis.

5.8 Fluid Resuscitation in Sepsis

Four phases of resuscitation in septic shock have been described—resuscitation, optimisation, stabilisation and evacuation (the ROSE model). In the early stage of septic shock, the patient enters the *ebb* phase of shock. There is vasodilation resulting in circulatory shock and arterial hypotension. Cardiac output can be high (hyperdynamic circulatory shock) or low. In this initial phase, resuscitation requires early adequate IV fluid resuscitation [3, 20]. The volume of fluid and markers of response to fluid resuscitation have been a matter of great debate. Previously, an algorithm for the resuscitation of patients with sepsis known as "early goal-directed therapy" (EGDT) was used [26]. The algorithm proposed in EGDT sought to provide haemodynamic targets to guide resuscitation efforts. The targets included a central venous pressure (CVP) of 8–12 mmHg, mean arterial pressure (MAP) of >65 mmHg and a central venous oxygen saturation (ScvO$_2$) of >70%. The goal was to normalise ScvO$_2$ within 6 hours in patients with septic shock using ongoing fluid boluses in combination with vasopressors. However, subsequent large multicentre randomised control trials compared EGDT to standard care and showed no outcome benefit in the EGDT arms of the trials, with increased volumes of fluids in the EGDT arms of the trials, and increased hospitalisation costs (Tables 5.3 and 5.4) [8]. The 2016 SSC guidelines removed ScvO$_2$ targets in light of these results [4], and resuscitation on the basis of ScvO$_2$ targets is no longer recommended.

However, there is a role for the measurement of ScvO$_2$ in the assessment of the patient undergoing resuscitation. A low ScvO$_2$ (<70%) indicates that oxygen delivery (DO$_2$) is compromised requiring measures to increase cardiac output (further fluid boluses or positive inotropes/chronotropes) unless haemoglobin concentrations are low (when transfusion to increase oxygen carrying capacity of blood would be an appropriate intervention). A high ScvO$_2$ (>80%) in septic shock can be interpreted that attempts to increase DO$_2$ are not going to improve the clinical picture [39]. Of course, ScvO$_2$ should not be measured in isolation; it should be part of the clinical assessment along with mean arterial pressure, central venous pressure, lactate, base deficit, strong ion difference, and markers of end organ perfusion such as urine output.

Table 5.3 Overview of studies on goal-directed therapy

Author	Year	Ref	n	Setting	Mortality EGDT	Mortality control
Rivers	2001	[26]	263	ER	38/130 (29.2%)	59/133 (44.4%)
Wang	2006	[27]	33	NA	4/16 (25%)	7/17 (41.2%)
De Oliveira[a]	2008	[28]	102	mixed	6/51 (11.8%)	20/51 (39.2%)
EGDT	2010	[29]	314	NA	41/163 (25.2%)	64/151 (42.4%)
LACTATE	2010	[30]	348	ICU	58/171 (33.9%)	77/177 (43.5%)
Jones	2010	[31]	300	ER	34/150 (22.7%)	25/150 (16.7%)
Tian	2012	[32]	71	NA	12/19 (63.2%)	12/34 (35.3%)
Yu	2013	[33]	50	NA	6/23 (26.1%)	5/25 (20%)
Lu	2014	[34]	82	NA	7/40 (17.5%)	7/42 (16.7%)
PROCESS	2014	[35]	1341	ER	92/439 (21%)	167/902 (18.5%)
SEPSISPAM	2014	[36]	776	ICU	142/388 (36.6%)	132/388 (34%)
ARISE	2014	[37]	1600	ER	147/792 (18.6%)	150/796 (18.8%)
PROMISE	2015	[38]	1260	ER	184/623 (29.5%)	181/620 (29.2%)
Total			*6491*		*771/3005 (25.7%)*	*906/3486 (26%)*

EGDT early goal-directed therapy, *ER* emergency room, *ICU* intensive care unit, *NA* not available, *n* number of patients included. Table adapted from Vandervelden et al. with permission (Open access CC BY 4.0 Licence) [8]
[a]Paediatric patients from ER, ward and ICU

Table 5.4 Effect of EGDT on mortality in patients presenting to the emergency room or ICU with septic shock. Primary mortality outcome is given for each study. The control was usual care or another non-EGDT resuscitation strategy. Fixed-effect model: the individual points denote the OR of each study and the lines either side the 95% confidence intervals. *OR* odds ratio, *CI* confidence interval. Table adapted from Vandervelden et al. with permission (Open access CC BY 4.0 Licence) [8]

Study or subgroup	EGDT		Control		Weight	Odds ratio M-H, Fixed, 95% CI	Odds ratio M-H, Fixed, 95% CI
	Events	Total	Events	Total			
ARISE investigators (2014)	147	792	150	796	19.8%	0.98 [0.76, 1.26]	
de Oliveira (2008)	6	51	20	51	2.9%	0.21 [0.07, 0.57]	
EGDT collaborative group (2010)	41	163	64	151	8.1%	0.46 [0.28, 0.74]	
Jones (2010)	34	150	25	150	3.1%	1.47 [0.82, 2.60]	
LACTATE study group (2010)	58	171	77	177	8.1%	0.67 [0.43, 1.03]	
Lu (2014)	7	40	7	42	0.9%	1.06 [0.34, 3.35]	
PROCESS Investigators (2014)	92	439	167	902	14.0%	1.17 [0.88, 1.55]	
P ROMISE Investigators (2015)	184	623	181	620	20.8%	1.02 [0.80, 1.30]	
Rivers (2001)	38	130	59	133	6.7%	0.52 [0.31, 0.86]	
SEPSISPAM Investigators (2014)	142	388	132	388	13.6%	1.12 [0.83, 1.50]	
Tian (2012)	12	19	12	34	0.5%	3.14 [0.98, 10.10]	
Wang (2006)	4	16	7	17	0.8%	0.48 [0.11, 2.11]	
Yu (2013)	6	23	5	25	0.6%	1.41 [0.37, 5.45]	
Total (95% CI)		*3005*		*3486*	*100.0%*	*0.94 [0.84, 1.05]*	
Total events	771		906				

Heterogeneity Chi² = 36.51, df = 12 (*P* = 0.0003) *I*² = 67%

Test for overall effect: *Z* = 1.11 (*P* = 0.27)

In the optimisation stage of fluid therapy in septic shock, the key clinical question is at which point should fluid therapy be stopped to avoid the complications associated with volume overload. Dynamic indices of fluid responsiveness (PPV, SVV, passive leg raise, etc.) should be monitored on an ongoing basis. Evidence that the patient has stopped being fluid responsive should prompt a cessation in IV fluid administration. Measurement of serial lactate levels is an established method of guiding resuscitation in shock states and is included in sepsis guidelines. A decrease in lactate is associated with better clinical outcomes, and is not just an association limited to patients with sepsis [40]. However, de-escalation of fluid resuscitation should be considered even before hyperlactataemia resolves. Lactate metabolism is not linear and exhibits two-phase kinetics. The early reduction in lactate concentration during the first 6 h of resuscitation is considered to be flow-responsive hyperlactataemia and represents improvement in perfusion and oxygen delivery to tissues. Hyperlactataemia persisting after perfusion is restored is flow-independent hyperlactataemia and relates to reduction in lactate clearance rather than lactate production by hypoperfused tissues (especially liver). Therefore, resuscitation with fluids should not persist until lactate levels normalise [41].

As discussed, overly aggressive IV fluid resuscitation in the treatment of hypotension or hyperlactataemia in sepsis can result in over-resuscitation. Fluid resuscitation induced vasodilation can result in decompensation of the arterial side of the circulation, resulting in higher vasopressor requirements. This may be as a result of blunting of baroreceptor-reflex mediated vasoconstriction in response to prevailing hypovolaemia, recruitment of previously collapsed vessels, as well as shear stress related endothelial nitric oxide (NO) release resulting in vasodilation [42]. Liberal fluid resuscitation has been shown to cause increased morbidity and mortality in children [14].

There have been no large randomised control trials in adults looking specifically at the effects of liberal versus restrictive fluid volumes during the initial resuscitation with sepsis and septic shock, although several are ongoing. However, it has been shown that achievement of a negative fluid balance is associated with better outcomes, and that volume overload leads to poorer outcomes in septic patients [11]. Large volume fluid resuscitation results in tissue oedema, impairing oxygen diffusion, and compromising blood flow in encapsulated organs and may lead to global increased permeability syndrome. In addition, large volume resuscitation increases intra-abdominal pressure and can cause abdominal compartment syndrome [11]. A balance needs to be struck between the needs of restoring circulating volume in the initial acute phase (ebb phase), and selecting an appropriate point at which a more restrictive fluid strategy is then instituted (flow phase). As it stands, there are few gold standard methods to determine when the resuscitation phase is completed but the absence of fluid responsiveness or a negative passive leg raise test can be helpful [3].

The stabilisation phase follows the optimisation phase, and occurs over days, and is characterised by the resolution of shock. The patient is in steady state, and IV fluid therapy should only be given as maintenance to replace normal losses (renal, insensible, gastrointestinal) and/or replacement of ongoing losses as a result of unresolved pathological conditions. The fourth phase is evacuation in which patients enter the *flow* phase with spontaneous evacuation of excess fluids, or in some critically ill patient, there may be ongoing global increased permeability syndrome. De-resuscitation occurs in this phase, with transition to negative fluid balance, either through the use of diuretics or renal replacement therapy with net negative ultrafiltration. Overly aggressive fluid removal carries the risk of inducing hypovolaemia, haemodynamic deterioration and hypoperfusion. Use of the tools described (PPV, SVV, passive leg raise, TTE, etc.) can help to identify the point at which the patient has become fluid responsive again, at which point fluid removal strategies should be de-escalated [3].

5.9 Vasoactive Agents

As described above, vasopressors and positively inotropic drugs are commonly required in resuscitation of the shocked patient. They can be classified into two general groups: the catecholamines and non-catecholamines. Endogenous catecholamines include adrenaline, noradrenaline and dopamine, while synthetic sympathomimetic drugs include phenylephrine and dobutamine. The non-catecholamine drugs include vasopressin receptor agonists (vasopressin), calcium-sensitising agents (e.g. levosimendan) and phosphodiesterase inhibitors (e.g. milrinone). The effects of vasoactive drugs on pressure and flow of blood in the various circulatory systems in the body (renal, mesenteric, etc.) are related to the relative distribution of receptors such as the α_1 and β_2 adrenoceptors.

The catecholamine drugs are agonists at α_1, β_1 and β_2 adrenoceptors, as well as dopamine receptors (D_1–D_5). Agonism of the α_1 adrenoceptor causes smooth muscle contraction in the vasculature resulting in increased systemic vascular resistance and an increased arterial blood pressure. The β_1 adrenoceptor is located in the heart and agonism at this receptor results in increased myocardial contractility (positive inotropy) and increased heart rate (positive chronotropy). The β_2 adrenoceptor is found throughout the systemic vasculature and stimulation causes smooth muscle relaxation and a fall in systemic vascular resistance. Dopamine receptors are found in the kidneys and brain. Stimulation of renal dopaminergic receptors causes a decrease in vascular resistance in the renal and mesenteric via vasodilation. Vasopressin analogues act at the V_1 (causing systemic, renal, splanchnic and coronary vasoconstriction), V_2 (causing antidiuresis at the level of the renal tubule) and V_3 receptors (causing ACTH secretion from the anterior pituitary).

- *Noradrenaline* is the vasopressor of choice in septic shock [4]. It has predominant α_1 activity with some β_1 and β_2 activity at higher dose. It causes peripheral vasoconstriction, increased myocardial contractility and increased heart rate. Its side effects include cardiac arrhythmias and peripheral ischaemia.
- *Adrenaline* also has activity at α_1, β_1 and β_2 adrenoceptors, but exhibits more dose-related effects. It has more predominant β adrenoceptor effects at lower doses causing increased myocardial contractility and increased heart rate. At

higher doses it has potent α_1 activity. Side effects of adrenaline infusion include cardiac arrhythmias, peripheral ischaemia, lactic acidosis and decreased splanchnic blood flow.

- *Dopamine* is a precursor of noradrenaline and adrenaline, as well as having intrinsic vasoactive properties. It is an agonist at α_1 and β_1 adrenoceptors, as well as dopamine receptors D1 to D5. It increases myocardial contractility, increases heart rate and causes peripheral vasoconstriction. It also causes renal and mesenteric vasodilation. At low doses its renal and mesenteric vasodilatory properties predominate, and as doses increase its β_1 effects emerge. At high doses, its α_1 effects are seen. It is associated with atrial and ventricular tachyarrhythmias. Its preferable effects on the splanchnic circulation compared to adrenaline and noradrenaline in septic shock would make it a good choice in the septic general surgical patient; however, its use is typically restricted to use in those with septic shock with bradycardia [43].

- *Vasopressin*, also known as antidiuretic hormone, is an endogenous hormone secreted from the posterior pituitary. When given as an infusion in shock, agonism at the V_1 receptor causes vasoconstriction. It also causes sensitization to catecholamines. It is usually used as a second-line vasopressor when escalating doses of noradrenaline are required for the treatment of refractory shock. It is associated with bradycardia, cardiac arrhythmias, bronchoconstriction, decreased splanchnic blood flow, and ischaemia and necrosis of tissues at high doses.

5.10   Coagulopathy and DIC in the Septic Surgical Patient

Sepsis is a common cause of disseminated intravascular coagulation (DIC), which produces a thrombotic coagulopathy. There is widespread microvascular thrombosis with a consumption of platelets, fibrinogen and clotting factors, which then results in bleeding. It may be occult or overt and is recognised clinically as bruising, epistaxis, oozing around catheter insertion sites, or overt haemorrhage. Routine laboratory results show derangement in the prothrombin time (PT) and activated partial thromboplastin time (aPTT) as a result of clotting factor consumption. There is a reduction in fibrinogen levels and a reduced platelet count. Fragmentocytes may be present.

The mainstay of management of DIC is treatment of the provoking cause. Daily or twice daily assessment of the patients clotting status should be made. In the emergency surgical patient with suspected DIC, platelets should be transfused to a level of $>50 \times 10^9/L$ and clotting factors should be replaced in the form of cryoprecipitate or fresh frozen plasma (FFP). Ongoing FFP transfusions may be required. Treatment should be individualised and under the guidance of a haematologist [44].

5.11   Conclusion

Due to the complexity of modern healthcare management of critically ill patients, the team approach to emergency surgery care is crucial to optimise surgical outcomes. Advances in management of critically patients from both a critical care and surgical standpoint have meant surgery is being offered to patients whose critical illness may have previously been a barrier to surgical intervention. Resuscitation is among the first steps in the patient journey, and when done well, can have a major influence on improving patient outcomes. The corollary is also true. Significant morbidity and mortality is associated with over-resuscitation of patients with IV fluids, delays to provision of antibiotics, and inadequate source control. It is imperative that a team approach is taken in management of these complex patients and principles of good resuscitative care and good IV fluid stewardship are observed from the outset.

Acknowledgement and Conflict of Interest Dr. Manu Malbrain is professor at the faculty of Medicine and Pharmacy at the Vrije Universiteit Brussels (VUB) and member of the Executive Committee of the Abdominal Compartment Society, formerly known as the World Society of Abdominal Compartment Syndrome (https://www.wsacs.org/). He is inaugural President and co-founder of WSACS and current Treasurer. He is co-founder of the International Fluid Academy (IFA). The IFA is integrated within the not-for-profit charitable organisation iMERiT, International Medical Education and Research Initiative, under Belgian law. The content of the IFA website (http://www.fluid academy.org) is based on the philosophy of FOAM (Free Open Access Medical education – #FOAMed). The site recently received the HONcode quality label for medical education (https://www.healthonnet.org/HONcode/Condu ct.html?HONConduct519739). He is a member of the Medical Advisory Board of Pulsion Medical Systems (now fully integrated in Getinge, Solna, Sweden) and Serenno Medical (Tel Aviv, Israel), consults for Baxter, Maltron, ConvaTec, Acelity, Spiegelberg and Holtech Medical.

References

1. Van der Mullen J, Wise R, Vermeulen G, Moonen PJ, Malbrain M. Assessment of hypovolaemia in the critically ill. Anaesthesiol Intensive Ther. 2018;50(2):141–9. https://doi.org/10.5603/AIT.a2017.0077.
2. Vincent JL, De Backer D. Circulatory shock. N Engl J Med. 2013;369:1726–43. https://doi.org/10.1056/NEJMra1208943.
3. Malbrain MLNG, Van Regenmortel N, Saugel B, De Tavernier B, Van Gaal P-J, Joannes-Boyau O, et al. Principles of fluid management and stewardship in septic shock: it is time to consider the four D's and the four phases of fluid therapy. Ann Intensive Care. 2018;8(1):66. https://doi.org/10.1186/s13613-018-0402-x.
4. Rhodes A, Evans LE, Alhazzani W, Levy MM, Antonelli M, Ferrer R, et al. Surviving sepsis campaign: international guidelines for management of sepsis and septic shock: 2016. Intensive Care Med. 2017;43(3):304–77. https://doi.org/10.1007/s00134-017-4683-6.
5. Finfer S, Myburgh J, Bellomo R. Intravenous fluid therapy in critically ill adults. Nat Rev Nephrol. 2018;14(9):541–57. https://doi.org/10.1038/s41581-0044-0.
6. Milford EM, Reade MC. Resuscitation fluid choices to preserve the endothelial glycocalyx. In: Vincent JL, editor. Annual update in intensive care and emergency medicine 2019. New York: Springer; 2019. p. 259–76. https://doi.org/10.1007/978-3-030-06067-1.

7. Jacobs R, Lochy S, Malbrain MLNG. Phenylephrine-induced recruitable preload from the venous side. J Clin Monit Comput. 2018;33(3):373–6. https://doi.org/10.1007/s10877-018-0225-1.
8. Vandervelden S, Malbrain ML. Initial resuscitation from severe sepsis: one size does not fit all. Anaesthesiol Intensive Ther. 2015;47 Spec no:s44–55. https://doi.org/10.5603/AIT.a2015.0075.
9. Verbrugge FH, Dupont M, Steels P, Grieten L, Malbrain M, Tang WHW, et al. Abdominal contributions to cardiorenal dysfunction in congestive heart failure. J Am Coll Cardiol. 2013;62(6):485–95. https://doi.org/10.1016/j.jacc.2013.04.070.
10. Malbrain ML, Roberts DJ, Sugrue M, De Keulenaer BL, Ivatury R, Pelosi P, et al. The polycompartment syndrome: a concise state-of-the-art review. Anaesthesiol Intensive Ther. 2014;46(5):433–50. https://doi.org/10.5603/AIT.2014.0064.
11. Malbrain ML, Marik PE, Witters I, Cordemans C, Kirkpatrick AW, Roberts DJ, et al. Fluid overload, de-resuscitation, and outcomes in critically ill or injured patients: a systematic review with suggestions for clinical practice. Anaesthesiol Intensive Ther. 2014;46(5):361–80. https://doi.org/10.5603/AIT.2014.0060.
12. Kirkpatrick AW, Roberts DJ, De Waele J, Jaeschke R, Malbrain M, De Keulenaer B, et al. Intra-abdominal hypertension and the abdominal compartment syndrome: updated consensus definitions and clinical practice guidelines from the World Society of the Abdominal Compartment Syndrome. Intensive Care Med. 2013;39(7):1190–206. https://doi.org/10.1007/s00134-013-2906-z.
13. Spahn DR, Bouillon B, Cerny V, Duranteau J, Filipescu D, Hunt BJ, et al. The European guideline in management of major bleeding and coagulopathy following trauma; fifth edition. Crit Care. 2019;23:98. https://doi.org/10.1186/s13054-019-2347-3.
14. Maitland K, George EC, Evans JA, Kiguli S, Olupot-Olupot P, Akech SO, et al. Exploring mechanisms of excess mortality with early fluid resuscitation: insights from the FEAST trial. BMC Med. 2013;11:68. https://doi.org/10.1186/1741-7015-11-68.
15. Duchesne JC, Kaplan LJ, Balogh ZJ, Malbrain ML. Role of permissive hypotension, hypertonic resuscitation and the global increased permeability syndrome in patients with severe hemorrhage: adjuncts to damage control resuscitation to prevent intra-abdominal hypertension. Anaesthesiol Intensive Ther. 2015;47(2):143–55. https://doi.org/10.5603/AIT.a2014.0052.
16. Wise R, Faurie M, Malbrain MLNG, Hodgson E. Strategies for intravenous fluid resuscitation in trauma patients. World J Surg. 2017;41:1170–83. https://doi.org/10.1007/s00268-016-3865-7.
17. Odutayo A, Desborough MJR, Trivella M, Stanley AJ, Dorée C, Collins GS, et al. Restrictive versus liberal blood transfusion for gastrointestinal bleeding; a systematic review and meta-analysis of randomised control trials. Lancet Gastroenterol Hepatol. 2017;2:354–60. https://doi.org/10.1016/S2468-1253(17)30054-7.
18. Singer M, Deutschman CS, Seymour CW, Shankar-Hari M, Annane D, Bauer M, et al. The third international consensus definitions for sepsis and septic shock (Sepsis-3). JAMA. 2016;315(8):801–10. https://doi.org/10.1001/jama.2016.0287.
19. Rhodes A, Philips G, Beale R, Cecconi M, Chiche JD, De Backer D, et al. The surviving sepsis campaign bundles and outcome: results from the international multicenter prevalence study on sepsis (the IMPreSS study). Intensive Care Med. 2015;41(9):1620–8. https://doi.org/10.1007/s00134-015-3906-y.
20. Levy MM, Evans LE, Rhodes A. The surviving sepsis campaign bundle: 2018 update. Crit Care Med. 2018;46(6):997–1000. https://doi.org/10.1097/CCM.0000000000003119.
21. Levy MM, Fink MP, Marshall JC, Abraham E, Angus D, Cook D, et al. 2001 SCCM/ESICM/ACCP/ATS/SIS International sepsis definitions conference. Intensive Care Med. 2003;29:530–8. https://doi.org/10.1007/s00134-003-1662-x.
22. Vincent JL, Moreno R, Takala J, Willatts S, De Mendonça A, Bruining H, et al. Working group on sepsis-related problems of the European society of intensive care medicine. The SOFA (sepsis-related organ failure assessment score to describe organ dysfunction/failure). Intensive Care Med. 1996;22(7):707–10. https://doi.org/10.1007/BF01709751.

23. National Institute of Health and Care Excellence. Surgical site infections: prevention and treatment (NICE guideline 125). 2019. https://nice.org.uk/guidance/ng125. Accessed 08 May 2019.
24. Kumar A, Roberts D, Wood KE, Light B, Parrillo JE, Sharma S, et al. Duration of hypotension before initiation of effective antimicrobial therapy is the critical determinant of survival in human septic shock. Crit Care Med. 2006;34(6):1589–96. https://doi.org/10.1097/01. CCM.000217961.75225.E9.
25. Pupelis G, Drozdova N, Mukans M, Malbrain ML. Serum procalcitonin is a sensitive marker for septic shock and mortality in secondary peritonitis. Anaesthesiol Intensive Ther. 2014;46(4):262–73. https://doi.org/10.5603/AIT.2014.0043.
26. Rivers E, Nguyen B, Havstad S, Ressler J, Muzzin A, Knoblich B, et al. Early goal-directed therapy in the treatment of severe sepsis and septic shock. N Engl J Med. 2001;345:1368–77. https://doi.org/10.1056/NEJMoa010307.
27. Wang XZ, Lu CJ, Gao FQ, Li XH, Yan WF, Ning FY. Efficacy of goal-directed therapy in the treatment of septic shock. Zhongguo Wei Zhong Bing Ji Jiu Yi Xue. 2006;18:661–4.
28. De Oliveira CF, De Oliveira DS, Gottschald AF, Moura JD, Costa GA, Ventura AC, et al. ACCM/PALS haemodynamic support guidelines for paediatric septic shock: an outcomes comparison with and without monitoring central venous oxygen saturation. Intensive Care Med. 2008;34(6):1065–75. https://doi.org/10.1007/s00134-008-1085-9.
29. Early Goal-Directed Therapy Collaborative Group of Zhejiang Province. The effect of early goal-directed therapy on treatment of critical patients with severe sepsis/septic shock; a multicenter, prospective, randomised, controlled study. Zhongguo Wei Zhong Bing Ji Jiu Yi Xue. 2010;24:42–5.
30. Jansen TC, van Bommel J, Schoonderbeek FJ, Sleeswijk Visser SJ, van der Klooster JM, Lima AP, et al. Early lactate-guided therapy in intensive care unit patients: a multicentre, open-label, randomised control trial. Am J Respir Crit Care Med. 2010;1182(6):752–61. https://doi.org/10.1164/rccm.200912-1918OC.
31. Jones AE, Shapiro NI, Trzeciak S, Arnold RC, Claremont HA, Kline JA. Lactate clearance vs central venous oxygen saturation as goals of early sepsis therapy: a randomised clinical trial. JAMA. 2010;303:739–46. https://doi.org/10.1001/jama.2010.158.
32. Tian HH, Han SS, Lv CJ, Wang T, Li Z, Hao D, et al. The effect of early goal lactate clearance rate on the outcome of septic shock patients with severe pneumonia. Zhongguo Wei Zhong Bing Ji Jiu Yi Xue. 2012;24(1):42–5.
33. Yu B, Tian HY, Hu ZJ, Zhao C, Liu LX, Zhang Y, et al. Comparison of the effect of fluid resuscitation as guided either by lactate clearance rate or by central venous oxygen saturation in patients with sepsis. Zhongguo Wei Zhong Bing Ji Jiu Yi Xue. 2013;25(10):578–83. https://doi.org/10.3760/cma.j.issn.2095-4352.2013.10.002.
34. Lu N, Zheng R, Lin H, Shao J, Yu J. Clinical studies of surviving sepsis bundles according to PiCCO on septic shock patients. Zhongguo Wei Zhong Bing Ji Jiu Yi Xue. 2014;26:23–7. https://doi.org/10.3760/cma.j.issn.2095-4352.2014.01.005.
35. The ProCESS Investigators, Yealy DM, Kellum JA, Huang DT, Barnato AE, Weissfeld LA, et al. A randomised trial of protocol-based care for early septic shock. N Engl J Med. 2014;370(18):1683–93. https://doi.org/10.1056/NEJMoa1401602.
36. Asfar P, Meziani F, Hamel JF, Grelon F, Megarbane B, Anguel N, et al. High versus low blood-pressure target in patients with septic shock. N Engl J Med. 2014;370(17):1583–93. https://doi.org/10.1056/NEJMoa1312173.
37. ARISE Investigators, ANZICS, Clinical Trials Group, Peake SL, Delaney A, Baliey M, Bellomo R, et al. Goal-directed resuscitation for patients with early septic shock. N Engl J Med. 2014;371(16):1496–506. https://doi.org/10.1056/NEJMoa1404380.
38. Mouncey PR, Osborn TM, Power GS, Harrison DA, Sadique MZ, Grieve RD, et al. Trial of early, goal-directed resuscitation for septic shock. N Engl J Med. 2015;372(14):1301–11. https://doi.org/10.1056/NEJMoa1500896.
39. Teboul JL, Monnet X, De Backer D. Should we abandon measuring SvO_2 or $ScvO_2$ in patients with sepsis? In: Vincent JL, editor. Annual update in intensive care and emergency medicine 2019. New York: Springer; 2019. p. 231–8. https://doi.org/10.1007/978-3-030-06067-1.

40. Vincent JL, Quintairos E Silva A, Couto L Jr, Taccone FS. The value of blood lactate kinetics in critically ill patients: a systematic review. Crit Care. 2016;20(1):257. https://doi.org/10.1186/s13054-016-1403-5.
41. Greco M, Messina A, Cecconi M. Lactate in critically ill patients: at the crossroads between perfusion and metabolism. In: Vincent JL, editor. Annual update in intensive care and emergency medicine 2019. New York: Springer; 2019. p. 199–211. https://doi.org/10.1007/978-3-030-06067-1.
42. Van Haren F, Byrne L, Litton E. Potential harm related to fluid resuscitation in sepsis. In: Vincent JL, editor. Annual update in intensive care and emergency medicine 2019. New York: Springer; 2019. p. 547–57.
43. De Backer D, Creteur J, Silva E, Vincent JL. Effects of dopamine, norepinephrine, and epinephrine on the splanchnic circulation in septic shock: which is best? Crit Care Med. 2003;31(6):1659–67. https://doi.org/10.1097/01.CCM.0000063045.77339.B6.
44. Squizzato A, Hunt BJ, Kinasewitz GT, Wada H, Ten Cate H, Thachil J, et al. Supportive management strategies for disseminated intravascular coagulation. An international consensus. Thromb Haemost. 2016;115(5):896–904. https://doi.org/10.1160/TH15-09-0740.

Medical Laboratory Support for Emergency Surgery

6

Maurice O'Kane

6.1 Introduction

The clinical management of the emergency surgery patient may be challenging and require the integration of clinical findings with the results from both laboratory testing and medical imaging. Clinical assessment may be confounded by the presence of co-morbid conditions (e.g. diabetes mellitus, chronic kidney disease, atherosclerotic vascular disease), the presence of which complicates both diagnosis and management.

The role of the laboratory is to offer a suitable repertoire of tests and provide results in a timely manner to support the clinical assessment and management of patients. The repertoire of tests provided should also include those relevant to any of the commonly occurring co-morbid conditions. The laboratory disciplines principally involved in the *acute setting* include clinical biochemistry, haematology/blood bank and medical microbiology although rarely support from other laboratory disciplines may also be required, e.g. immunology. The value of a laboratory test lies in its ability to provide information that contributes to the diagnosis or stratification of patients.

A useful *diagnostic* test is one that has high sensitivity and specificity for ruling in or ruling out a particular condition. In patients presenting with acute abdominal pain, it is rarely the case that any single laboratory test has sufficient sensitivity or specificity to allow a 'rule in' or 'rule out' decision on its own. Even the best performing of the commonly requested tests in emergency surgery patients, amylase and lipase, have a sub-optimal performance with diagnostic sensitivity of 90.3–93%

M. O'Kane (✉)
Clinical Chemistry Laboratory, Altnagelvin Hospital, Western Health and Social Care Trust, Londonderry, Northern Ireland, UK
e-mail: Maurice.OKane@westerntrust.hscni.net

© World Society of Emergency Surgery and Donegal Clinical and Research Academy 2020   51
M. Sugrue et al. (eds.), *Resources for Optimal Care of Emergency Surgery*,
Hot Topics in Acute Care Surgery and Trauma,
https://doi.org/10.1007/978-3-030-49363-9_6

and a specificity of 78.7–92.6% respectively for the diagnosis of acute pancreatitis [1]. Most of the commonly requested tests in emergency surgery patients, e.g. liver enzymes such as ALT or GGT, lack diagnostic specificity and may be abnormal in a range of conditions. It is more usually the case that laboratory tests provide information that helps narrow down a differential diagnosis [2]. In patients presenting with non-traumatic abdominal pain, a combination of diagnostic and imaging tests changed the likely diagnosis in 37% of subjects [3].

Laboratory tests also provide information that allows patient *stratification*. For example, C-reactive protein (CRP) concentration is used in the assessment of severity of inflammatory response and plasma lactate concentration in the assessment of the severity of sepsis. Laboratory test results may be incorporated into scoring algorithms for patient assessment, e.g. the Sequential [Sepsis related] Organ Failure Assessment Score (SOFA) [4].

With increasing life expectancy in developed countries, the proportion of very elderly patients presenting to emergency surgery is increasing and such patients have high levels of co-morbidity: in the over 85 years population >90% have one or more co-morbidities, principally hypertension, respiratory disease, diabetes mellitus, hypothyroidism, heart failure and chronic kidney disease, all of which may impact on surgical diagnosis and management [5]. Laboratory test results play an essential role in the acute assessment of many of these conditions.

Clinical guidelines have not been prescriptive about the exact repertoire of tests required for the optimum management of emergency surgery patients. However, the following array of tests are commonly provided on a 24/7 basis: electrolytes, urea and creatinine, liver enzymes and bilirubin, amylase and/or lipase, calcium (including adjusted calcium), albumin, magnesium, CRP, cardiac troponin, blood gases, lactate, full blood count, dipstick urinalysis, serum or urine hCG, glucose, ethanol, coagulation testing, blood culture, wound culture, antimicrobial sensitivity . It may rarely be the case that other less routine tests are needed on an emergency basis, e.g. urine porphobilinogen and porphyrin measurement for the diagnosis of an acute porphyria, vasculitis screen and toxicology.

An emergency surgery service also has a requirement for the availability of blood and blood products.

6.2 Organization of Laboratory Services

Testing may be provided by a central laboratory but increasingly many tests are also now available at point-of-care (see below).

A key attribute of good collaborative working between laboratory and clinical teams is excellent communication. There should be agreement as to the repertoire of tests to be provided (including which tests should be available at point-of-care) and the turnaround time for reporting results. Senior laboratory staff should be available, as necessary to provide advice on appropriate test selection and interpretation of results where necessary and on the choice of antimicrobial regimens.

Clinical staff should be aware that reference intervals for commonly requested tests may vary between laboratories depending on the specific commercial assay used; this is particularly the case for enzyme activity measurements (e.g. amylase and liver enzymes) and also analytes measured by immunoassay such as CRP, thyroid hormones or cortisol. In the case of CRP measurement, one widely used commercial immunoassay has a significant negative measurement bias compared to other commonly used assays. These differences have the potential to cause problems when using literature-derived algorithms for patient management which are based on different assays to those used in the local laboratory. In some cases, the reporting units for test results may vary between laboratories (even within the same country or region), e.g. PaO_2 /$PaCO_2$ reported in mmHg or kPa, Hb in mg/dL or mg/L or mmol/L and ethanol in mg/dL or mg /L. All this has the potential to cause confusion and patient harm and is especially relevant for new clinical staff who have previously worked elsewhere. It is therefore important that clinical staff familiarize themselves with the detail of the service provided by their local laboratory. Such information should be available in the laboratory handbook.

Given the essential role of the medical laboratory in patient care, it is important that services are delivered to a high standard. The International Organization for Standardization (ISO) document 'ISO 15189: 2012 Medical Laboratories—Requirement for quality and competence' defines the standards to which a medical laboratory service should be provided. This covers the full range of laboratory activities outlined under Management and Technical requirements. Compliance with the requirements of ISO 15189 provides assurance to users that the laboratory service is delivered to a high quality. Ideally compliance should be confirmed by a relevant national accrediting body. Individual countries may also have separate specific regulations and requirements for professional staff and activities. The supply and administration of blood products may be subject to national legislation and regulated by a designated national competent authority.

6.3 Point-of-Care Testing

A major advance in medical laboratory analytical technology over the last 20 years has been the development of small portable or benchtop analysers designed to be operated at the patient's bedside (point-of-care [POC]) by members of the clinical team. Removing the need to transport samples to a central laboratory allows a more rapidly available test result and offers the possibility of expediting clinical decision making.

POC analysers are now in widespread use for a broad repertoire of tests of relevance to emergency surgery patients and include: blood gas/electrolytes, glucose, lactate, hydroxybutyrate, creatinine, cardiac troponin, urine dipstick analysis, urine pregnancy testing, INR testing. There is an ever expanding array of more complex markers including sepsis panels, bacterial pathogen detection panels either currently available or under development.

POC analysers typically require very small sample volumes (venous, arterial, capillary blood or urine) and generate results within seconds or minutes. Unlike central laboratory testing which is performed by qualified laboratory analysts, POC instruments are designed for use by clinical staff and are engineered to ensure that instrument calibration, maintenance, sample processing and quality checks are easy and straightforward. Where possible POC instruments should allow electronic transmission of results to the laboratory information systems and/or the patient electronic record to ensure permanent and retrievable documentation of POC test results.

The analytical performance of POC tests should be appropriate to clinical requirements. For some POC tests, analytical performance may be less good than the equivalent central laboratory assay, e.g. POC troponin may not have the same analytical performance as a high sensitivity laboratory troponin assay and this will impact on the diagnostic performance of the test. It is therefore important that the required analytical performance of a POC test is pre-specified and that delivery of this is verified for the instrument in question.

Despite the design features of POC instruments which offer ease and simplicity of use, there is evidence of a higher rate of quality errors when compared with central laboratory testing with an obvious potential to cause patient harm; for the most part these relate to operator error [6]. The POC service within a hospital is generally overseen by the central laboratory. The necessary quality framework is outlined in a further ISO document: 'POC: Point-of-care testing (POCT)—Requirements for Quality and Competence (ISO 22870:2016)'. This document used in conjunction with ISO 151892012 outlines the technical and managerial requirements for a POC service which include instrument evaluation and selection, clinical user protocols and procedures, training and certification of users. Ideally, compliance with the ISO 22870:2016 should be confirmed by a relevant national accrediting body.

References

1. Lameris W, van Randen A, van Es HW, et al. Imaging strategies for detection of urgent conditions in patients with acute abdominal pain: diagnostic accuracy study. BMJ. 2009;338:b2431.
2. Kristensen M, Iversen AKS, Gerds TA, et al. Routine blood tests are associated with short term mortality and can improve emergency department triage: a cohort study of >12,000 patients. Scand J Trauma Resus Emer Med. 2017;25:1–8.
3. Nagurney JT, Brown DFM, Chang Y, et al. Use of diagnostic testing in the emergency department for patients presenting with non-traumatic abdominal pain. J Emer Med. 2003;25:363–71.
4. Singer M, Deutschman CS, Warren Seymour C, et al. The third international consensus definitions for sepsis and septic shock (sepsis-3). JAMA. 2016;315:801–10.
5. Merani S, Payne J, Padwal RS, et al. Predictors of in-hospital mortality and complications in very elderly patients undergoing emergency surgery. World J Emer Surg. 2014;9:43.
6. O'Kane MJ, McManus P, McGowan N, Lynch PLM. Quality error rates in point-of-care testing. Clin Chem. 2011;57:1267–71.

Radiology and Emergency Surgery

7

Gavin Sugrue, Ruth M. Conroy, and Michael Sugrue

7.1   Introduction

Radiologists are key members of the multidisciplinary team and play an integral role in the diagnosis and management of patients pre- and post-emergency surgery. Through a timely and accurate diagnosis of potentially life-threatening conditions, radiological services facilitate the clinical decision-making process for appropriate surgical, interventional or conservative management. The ultimate goal is for radiology input to assist in optimising outcomes in patients requiring emergency surgical intervention.

Just as emergency surgical patients require appropriate access to surgical care [1], these acutely ill and injured patients require access to emergency imaging, both inside and outside conventional working hours. Thus, the increasing requirement for cross-sectional imaging around-the-clock and the need for radiologists to deliver contemporaneous reports have given rise to the emergency radiology subspecialty. To meet this demand, many large academic centres now provide 24/7 emergency radiology coverage [2], complete with in-house staff radiologists and radiology personnel.

G. Sugrue (✉)
Department of Radiology, Vancouver General Hospital, Vancouver, BC, Canada

R. M. Conroy
Department of Radiology, Altnagelvin Hospital, Derry, UK

M. Sugrue
Letterkenny University Hospital and University Hospital Galway,
Letterkenny, Donegal, Ireland

EU INTERREG Emergency Surgery Outcomes Advancement Project (eSOAP),
Letterkenny University Hospital, Letterkenny, Donegal, Ireland

© World Society of Emergency Surgery and Donegal Clinical and Research Academy 2020   55
M. Sugrue et al. (eds.), *Resources for Optimal Care of Emergency Surgery*,
Hot Topics in Acute Care Surgery and Trauma,
https://doi.org/10.1007/978-3-030-49363-9_7

7.2   Emergency Radiology: Logistics and Location

A radiology department must be structured and organised to allow for diagnostic evaluation of the acutely ill patient [3]. Increasing numbers of emergency radiology departments are co-located within the emergency department, which facilitates radiology's contribution to management of the emergency surgical patient. In particular, expedited imaging performed in acutely ill trauma patients within the first hour after trauma, termed "the golden hour", has been shown to improve survival [4]. Furthermore, utilisation of standardised radiological algorithms ensures that radiological decisions are made in the correct sequence and necessary time frame [5].

7.3   Emergency Radiology: Technology

Computed Tomography (CT) is the key imaging modality in the assessment of acutely ill patients. Rapid advances in CT technology allow for high quality rapid imaging to be performed [6]. CT has a higher sensitivity in diagnosing potentially life-threatening conditions than X-rays or point of care ultrasound, such as Focused Assessment with Sonography for Trauma (FAST) [7]. Thus many institutions have CT scanners based within the emergency department to expedite the imaging process. This is of particular benefit to patients not suitable for an intrahospital transfer to the radiology department [8]. However, despite these continued radiological advances, undertaking a CT study in a hemodynamically unstable patient presents significant challenges, often generating debate regarding its feasibility and potential benefit [9].

Artificial intelligence (AI), particularly deep learning, is a rapidly progressing field in radiology [10]. To date, radiologists have visually assessed images for the purpose of detection, characterisation and monitoring of disease. AI algorithms can detect complex patterns within imaging data-sets to assist radiologists in diagnosis [11]. Although not routinely used in clinical practice to date, AI has demonstrated promise in the assessment of lung cancer [12] and liver lesions [13] and will undoubtedly play an increasing role in imaging acutely ill patients in the future. For example, AI automated triaging of radiological studies is now possible. This may be of particular value in high volume emergency departments, with AI software prioritising "abnormal" cases to be reviewed by the radiologist prior to "normal" studies [14].

Over the past decade there has been a rapid rise in teleradiology [15], a service which transmits digitised patient images, such as X-rays, CTs, and MRIs, from one location to another for the purpose of interpretation. This service has helped many institutions overcome resource and geographical challenges, providing smaller hospitals with round-the-clock subspecialty coverage ensuring that there is no compromise in patient care [16].

7.4   Emergency Radiology: Imaging Protocols

Imaging studies are requested by a spectrum of healthcare providers who must be aware of the importance of adopting the correct imaging technique. By utilising the correct imaging protocol, the radiological study may be tailored to address a specific concern. For example, in a case of suspected mesenteric ischemia, a triphasic CT abdomen (non-contrast, arterial and portal venous phase study of abdomen and pelvis) is required to provide a detailed assessment [17]. No oral contrast is required. Failure to undertake bi- or triphasic abdominal imaging, or administration of oral contrast prior to CT acquisition, may reduce sensitivity for detection of signs of ischaemia in such a case. In a further example, the evaluation of a suspected gastro-intestinal bleed requires arterial and delayed phase imaging [18]. Non-contrast imaging is insufficient, and errors with incorrect CT protocols may directly result in reduced diagnostic accuracy, delay in diagnosis, excessive radiation, prolonged scanner time and increased cost. Hence clear communication between the radiologist and the referring clinician is essential regarding the suspected diagnosis or clinical question, combined with established institutional protocols, in order to avoid these pitfalls (Fig. 7.1).

Point of care ultrasound (PoCUS) is a diagnostic or procedural guidance ultrasound performed at the bedside by a clinician to guide patient management [19]. It acts as a complementary tool to traditional imaging modalities. The goals and

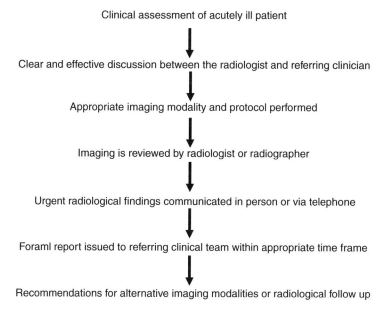

Fig. 7.1 Example of radiological workflow in imaging acutely ill patients

approach to the ultrasound are fundamentally different from a conventional departmental ultrasound, as it is limited to a specific clinical question without removing the patient from their clinical area, such as the trauma bay. For example, a FAST scan is used to assess for free fluid in the setting of trauma [20], detection of abdominal aortic aneurysm, thoracic ultrasound for pleural fluid detection and cardiac ultrasound for cardiac function evaluation [21].

7.5 Emergency Radiology: Education and Training

With the ultimate goal to improve patient care, it is essential to provide comprehensive training for junior radiologists. In many large academic centres, established residency and fellowship programmes, in conjunction with a consultant led service, provide valuable training. Dedicated fellowship programmes, specifically in emergency radiology, have been established to meet the increasing demand for imaging the acutely ill patient. Training focuses not only on the imaging manifestations of patients presenting to emergency departments and trauma centres, but seeks to find improvements in workflow management, protocolling and collaboration with emergency physicians and trauma care providers. Furthermore, for a radiology department to continue to provide a high standard of care, it is important for clear and effective communication, documentation, audit and peer review to exist, fostering strong relationships with key referring clinical services.

7.6 Emergency Radiology: Mass Casualty Incident

There is growing awareness of the need for hospitals to be prepared for a mass casualty incident (MCI) [22]. In an MCI, a significant number of injuries occur over a short period, often related to terrorism or natural disaster, often placing a significant strain on hospital resources. Many Level 1 trauma centres have recently established MCI protocols, which involve a multidisciplinary approach to manage a large influx of casualties [23]. Engagement of the radiology department in drawing up the MCI plans aims to maximise capacity and patient throughput, while at the same time minimising possible delays and errors, with the ultimate aim of reducing morbidity and mortality. Through careful planning and MCI drill training, MCI protocols aim to optimise future preparedness and outcomes.

7.7 Conclusion

Radiology departments play an integral role in the multidisciplinary management of emergency surgical patients. The development of the emergency radiology subspecialty, along with advances in technology and co-location of radiology facilities within emergency departments, aims to address the challenges of imaging patients in the emergency setting.

References

1. Hsee L, Devaud M, Middelberg L, Jones W, Civil I. Acute surgical unit at Auckland City Hospital: a descriptive analysis. ANZ J Surg. 2012;82(9):588–91.
2. Sellers A, Hillman BJ, Wintermark M. Survey of after-hours coverage of emergency department imaging studies by US academic radiology departments. J Am Coll Radiol. 2014;11(7):725–30.
3. Philipp MO, Kubin K, Hörmann M, Metz VM. Radiological emergency room management with emphasis on multidetector-row CT. Eur J Radiol. 2003;48(1):2–4.
4. Self ML, Blake AM, Whitley M, Nadalo L, Dunn E. The benefit of routine thoracic, abdominal, and pelvic computed tomography to evaluate trauma patients with closed head injuries. Am J Surg. 2003;186(6):609–14.
5. Linsenmaier U, Kanz KG, Rieger J, Rock C, Pfeifer KJ, Reiser M. Strukturierte radiologische Diagnostik beim Polytrauma. Radiologe. 2002;42(7):533–40.
6. Rubin GD. Computed tomography: revolutionizing the practice of medicine for 40 years. Radiology. 2014;273(2S):S45–74.
7. Deunk J, Dekker HM, Brink M, van Vugt R, Edwards MJ, van Vugt AB. The value of indicated computed tomography scan of the chest and abdomen in addition to the conventional radiologic work-up for blunt trauma patients. J Trauma Acute Care Surg. 2007;63(4):757–63.
8. Huber-Wagner S, Mand C, Ruchholtz S, Kühne CA, Holzapfel K, Kanz KG, et al. Effect of the localisation of the CT scanner during trauma resuscitation on survival—a retrospective, multicentre study. Injury. 2014;45:S76–82.
9. Tsutsumi Y, Fukuma S, Tsuchiya A, Ikenoue T, Yamamoto Y, Shimizu S, et al. Computed tomography during initial management and mortality among hemodynamically unstable blunt trauma patients: a nationwide retrospective cohort study. Scand J Trauma Resusc Emerg Med. 2017;25(1):74.
10. Wong SH, Al-Hasani H, Alam Z, Alam A. Artificial intelligence in radiology: how will we be affected? Eur Radiol. 2019;29(1):141–3.
11. Hosny A, Parmar C, Quackenbush J, Schwartz LH, Aerts HJ. Artificial intelligence in radiology. Nat Rev Cancer. 2018;17:1.
12. Coroller TP, Grossmann P, Hou Y, Velazquez ER, Leijenaar RT, Hermann G, et al. CT-based radiomic signature predicts distant metastasis in lung adenocarcinoma. Radiother Oncol. 2015;114(3):345–50.
13. Zhou LQ, Wang JY, Yu SY, Wu GG, Wei Q, Deng YB, et al. Artificial intelligence in medical imaging of the liver. World J Gastroenterol. 2019;25(6):672.
14. Tang A, Tam R, Cadrin-Chênevert A, Guest W, Chong J, Barfett J, et al. Canadian Association of Radiologists white paper on artificial intelligence in radiology. Canadian Assoc Radiol J. 2018;69(2):120–35.
15. https://www.acr.org/Practice-Management-Quality-Informatics/Legal-Practices/Teleradiology. Accessed April 2019.
16. Prabhakaran K, Lombardo G, Latifi R. Telemedicine for trauma and emergency management: an overview. Curr Trauma Reports. 2016;2(3):115–23.
17. Furukawa A, Kanasaki S, Kono N, Wakamiya M, Tanaka T, Takahashi M, et al. CT diagnosis of acute mesenteric ischemia from various causes. Am J Roentgenol. 2009;192(2):408–16.
18. Wells ML, Hansel SL, Bruining DH, Fletcher JG, Froemming AT, Barlow JM, et al. CT for evaluation of acute gastrointestinal bleeding. Radiographics. 2018;38(4):1089–107.
19. Moore CL, Copel JA. Point-of-care ultrasonography. N Engl J Med. 2011;364(8):749–57.
20. Kameda T, Taniguchi N. Overview of point-of-care abdominal ultrasound in emergency and critical care. J Intensive Care. 2016;4(1):53.
21. Koster G, van der Horst IC. Critical care ultrasonography in circulatory shock. Curr Opin Crit Care. 2017;23(4):326–33.

22. Berger FH, Körner M, Bernstein MP, Sodickson AD, Beenen LF, McLaughlin PD, et al. Emergency imaging after a mass casualty incident: role of the radiology department during training for and activation of a disaster management plan. Br J Radiol. 2016;89(1061):20150984.
23. Körner M, Geyer LL, Wirth S, et al. Analysis of responses of radiology personnel to a simulated mass casualty incident after the implementation of an automated alarm system in hospital emergency planning. Emerg Radiol. 2011;18:119–26. https://doi.org/10.1007/s10140-010-0922-7.

Interaction Between Gastroenterology and Emergency General Surgery

8

Chris Steele, Paula Loughlin, Angus Watson, and Michael Sugrue

8.1 Surgical Emergencies Associated with Gastroenterology

Emergency General Surgery involves the urgent care of admitted surgical emergencies and accounts for over 10% of all hospital admissions. In the USA alone, there are almost three million patients admitted for emergency gastrointestinal surgical problems and one-third of these will require surgery [1]. The commonest

C. Steele (✉)
Department of Gastroenterology, Letterkenny University Hospital,
Letterkenny, Co. Donegal, Ireland
e-mail: Chris.Steele@hse.ie

P. Loughlin
Department of Surgery, Altnagelvin Hospital, Derry-Londonderry, North Ireland, UK

EU INTERREG Centre for Personalised Medicine, Intelligent Systems Research Centre,
School of Computing, Engineering and Intelligent Systems, Ulster University,
Derry-Londonderry, North Ireland, UK
e-mail: Paula.Loughlin@westerntrust.hscni.net

A. Watson
EU INTERREG Centre for Personalised Medicine, Intelligent Systems Research Centre,
School of Computing, Engineering and Intelligent Systems, Ulster University,
Derry-Londonderry, North Ireland, UK

Raighmore Hospital, Inverness, Scotland, UK
e-mail: angus.watson@nhs.net

M. Sugrue (✉)
EU INTERREG Centre for Personalised Medicine, Intelligent Systems Research Centre,
School of Computing, Engineering and Intelligent Systems, Ulster University,
Derry-Londonderry, North Ireland, UK

Department of Surgery, Letterkenny University Hospital and Donegal Clinical Research
Academy, Letterkenny, Donegal, Ireland
e-mail: michael.sugrue@hse.ie

© World Society of Emergency Surgery and Donegal Clinical and Research Academy 2020   61
M. Sugrue et al. (eds.), *Resources for Optimal Care of Emergency Surgery*,
Hot Topics in Acute Care Surgery and Trauma,
https://doi.org/10.1007/978-3-030-49363-9_8

Table 8.1 Conditions
where gastroenterology
co-consultation is essential

1. Upper GI bleeding
2. Inflammatory bowel conditions
3. Peri-anal abscess and fistulation
4. Short bowel syndrome secondary to bowel resection
5. Gallstone pancreatitis

emergencies we see relate to cholecystitis, bowel obstruction, laparotomy, appendicitis and conditions that may be associated with GI bleeding, both upper and lower GI bleeding.

The team approach involving all disciplines will optimize outcome [2]. Gastroenterologists are fundamental to the management of patients with inflammatory bowel disease, ulcerative disease; both benign and malignant that bleeds and perforates [3, 4]. In addition, biliary disease with associated pancreatitis and subsequent intervention often requires the skill of gastroenterology.

Combined approaches with gastroenterology and surgeons are essential in the management of emergency inflammatory bowel admissions particularly to optimize medical therapy and come to a team decision when medical therapy fails.

Non-operative management of surgical emergencies occurs in two-thirds of patients. Gastroenterology should be involved in decision-making in many of the conditions as shown in Table 8.1.

Some patients may be admitted jointly, and some patients may be admitted directly under gastroenterologists. Involving gastroenterology in the Surgical Outcome Advancement Programmes of Emergency General Surgery is essential. An example of this is the Emergency Abdominal Surgery Course (EASC) where gastroenterologists are on the Faculty of the course. In addition, bleeding rosters around the world, while occasionally involving surgeons, generally utilize services of gastroenterology.

8.2 Conclusion

Interaction with gastroenterology and emergency general surgery is essential in the multi-disciplinary approach to optimize outcome.

References

1. Hernandez MC, Madbak F, Parikh K, Crandall M. GI surgical emergencies: scope and burden of disease. J Gastrointest Surg. 2019;23(4):827–36.
2. Symons NR, McArthur D, Miller A, Verjee A, Senapati A. Emergency general surgeons, subspeciality surgeons and the future management of emergency surgery: results of a national survey. Color Dis. 2019;21(3):342–8.
3. Alexakis C, Chhaya V, Sutherland I, Lalani R, Tavabie O, Hewett R, et al. PWE-128 the out-of-hours gastrointestinal bleed service in South-West London: a model for regional emergency endoscopy cover. Gut. 2016;65:A201.
4. Gibson R, Hitchcock K, Duggan AE. Characteristics of Australian after-hours emergency endoscopy services. J Gastroenterol Hepatol. 2006;21(3):569–71.

Advanced and Specialist Nursing Practice in Emergency Surgery: The Team Approach

9

Randal Parlour, Carol-Ann Walker, Louise Flanagan, and Paula Loughlin

9.1 Introduction

Increasingly we recognise the role of teamwork in the advancement of critical care across spectrums of both medicine and surgery. The unscheduled nature of critical illness and injury challenges surgical teams in the delivery of optimal patient care. Patients with emergency surgical conditions need prompt attention, early diagnosis and excellence in treatment to ensure good outcomes [1]. While there are a wide variety of patterns of presentation within emergency general surgery, seven key conditions account for in excess of 80.0% of all procedures, 80.3% of all deaths and 78.9% of all complications [2]. The development of optimum management for emergency general surgery conditions requires a dedicated multidisciplinary team approach. Such an approach fully acknowledges and supports the principle that successful care is based upon the contribution of various health professionals who advance the attainment of a successful outcome. This chapter will explore the role of advanced and specialist nursing practice as part of the team in emergency general surgery.

R. Parlour (✉)
EU INTERREG Emergency Surgery Outcomes Advancement Project (eSOAP),
Letterkenny University Hospital, Letterkenny, Co. Donegal, Ireland

Ulster University, Derry, Northern Ireland, UK
e-mail: Randal.Parlour@hse.ie

C.-A. Walker · L. Flanagan
Department of Surgery, EU INTERREG Emergency Surgery Outcomes Advancement Project
(eSOAP), Letterkenny University Hospital, Letterkenny, Co. Donegal, Ireland
e-mail: CarolAnn.Walker@hse.ie; Louise.Flanagan@hse.ie

P. Loughlin
Altnagelvin Hospital, Western Health & Social Care Trust,
Derry, Northern Ireland
e-mail: paula.loughlin@westerntrust.hscni.net

© World Society of Emergency Surgery and Donegal Clinical and Research Academy 2020   63
M. Sugrue et al. (eds.), *Resources for Optimal Care of Emergency Surgery*,
Hot Topics in Acute Care Surgery and Trauma,
https://doi.org/10.1007/978-3-030-49363-9_9

9.2   Advanced and Specialist Nursing Practice: Context

Internationally, advanced nursing practice roles have increased dramatically during the past 30–40 years. These roles initially evolved in Canada and the United States [3] and, during the past 20 years, have been developed across many European countries. Initially these roles were developed in response to a number of factors including: health service transformation; recognised service needs; a reduction in the working hours of junior doctors; and the opportunity for nurses to undertake advanced practice and deliver enhanced patient care and outcomes.

Role titles, scope of practice and role autonomy differ greatly depending upon the country in which advanced nursing practice is undertaken [4] and, in the past, this has inhibited an accepted definition. Nonetheless, there has been international agreement [5] on the core domains that underpin advanced nursing practice and these are: autonomy in clinical practice, expert practice, professional and clinical leadership and research.

The role of advanced nursing practice within an acute surgery environment has more recently been advocated within a number of strategic reports. In a report for The Nuffield Trust focusing upon challenges and opportunities in emergency general surgery [6], the introduction of advanced nurse practitioners (ANP) was proposed as a role that can make a significant impact on the quality of care delivered to EGS patients. Similarly, the Model of Care for Acute Surgery in Ireland [7] has recommended that ANP roles are established to support the role of medical clinicians particularly within emergency departments (ED) and acute surgical assessment units (ASAU).

9.3   Impact of Advanced and Specialist Nursing Practice: The Evidence

In a systematic review of the impact of advanced practice nursing roles on quality of care, clinical outcomes, patient satisfaction and cost in the emergency and critical care settings [8], a range of evidence was presented that has highlighted the positive impact attributed to these roles. It was reported [9] that advanced nursing practice enabled a more flexible model of service delivery based upon patient needs, while others [10, 11] reported positive effects of advanced nurse practitioners on clinical outcomes, patient satisfaction and costs.

A number of further significant metrics were also recognised [8]. In 'collaborative care involving advanced practice nurses' it was identified, from a trauma centre study [12], that a significantly shorter length of stay was associated with an advanced nurse practice physician collaboration. This was marked by greater communication with multidisciplinary teams, discharge planning, care coordination and administrative work and was enhanced by the competence of advanced nursing practitioners in these areas.

As regards patient mortality, it was further identified [8] that patients had lower ICU mortality under advanced nurse practice-directed care than those under physician-only care. Hospital mortality was similar between these groups in all of the studies reviewed. It was indicated that advanced practice nurses provided greater continuity of care within ICU as they were not subject to frequent rotation coverage as associated with junior physicians. As a consequence, advanced practice nurses were more conversant with the environment and patient needs than the physicians who were constantly on rotation. Advanced practice nurses were also considered to be a consistent point of contact for ICU staff and the multidisciplinary team. It has been previously indicated [13] that this leads to effective care coordination and improved patient outcomes. Overall, it has been concluded [8], from a synthesis of the available evidence across Australia, Canada, New Zealand, the UK and the USA, that advanced practice nurses appear to induce clinical outcomes commensurate with those of physicians in the emergency and critical care settings.

The positive impact of advanced nursing practitioners was also demonstrated within emergency care settings. Using important metrics associated with 'time from arrival to first assessment by physician' and 'time to treatment', it was considered that advanced nursing practitioners facilitated improved access to prompt emergency care and, in comparison with physicians, were observed to have greater adherence to the recommended targets for timely administration of analgesia [14].

A collective case study was undertaken [15] that evaluated the impact of ANP roles within an acute hospital including surgical settings. The findings evidently demonstrated that the ANPs had a positive impact on patient experience, patient outcomes and patient safety. Significantly, introduction of the ANPs also had a positive impact on other multidisciplinary staff members (Fig. 9.1) by enhancing knowledge, skills and competence along with less discernible measures, for example,

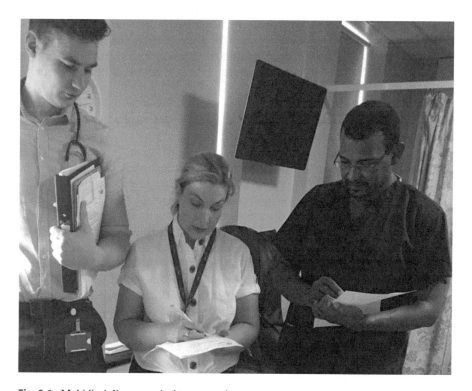

Fig. 9.1 Multidisciplinary surgical team members

quality of working life, distribution of workload and teamworking. It is noteworthy that the impact of ANP roles within these case studies was not intelligibly a direct outcome of delegating junior doctors' responsibilities, but was a consequence of advancements in care through implementation of a whole systems approach. These are clear examples of how ANPs were able to channel the efforts of the entire team in order to improve patient care and outcomes.

The role which advanced nursing practice can play in improving the care of laparotomy patients has recently been underlined [16]. This has been supported by the team at the National Emergency Laparotomy Audit (NELA) who have been central to advocating for increased nursing specialisation relevant to this patient group. It is anticipated that nursing expertise would be particularly effective in augmenting recovery and patients' overall experience of care.

Furthermore, the NELA team consider that specialist nurses could not only facilitate the timely collection of data for NELA audits but also enhance additional aspects of emergency surgical care including: transfer of patients to theatre in a timely fashion; post-operative administration of analgesia; recognition of deteriorating patients; ensuring continuity of care; provision of emotional support for patients and families and improving the patient experience.

The role that advanced practice nurses could play in the assessment process for emergency surgical care and in reducing post-operative complications has also been emphasised [16]. For example, in older patients, identification of undiagnosed cognitive impairment as early as possible is extremely important as it is directly related to post-operative delirium and to poorer outcomes. In these circumstances, it is considered that advanced practice nurses have the potential to make a positive impact on patient-reported outcomes and enable patients, at all stages of their surgical care, to take the decision that best accommodates their own individual needs.

9.4   Advanced and Specialist Surgical Nursing in Practice

The significance of understanding context in order to appreciate the manner in which 'evidence' and 'innovation' can influence practice has previously been asserted [17]. This outlined a multi-faceted approach comprising culture, leadership and evaluation in organisations, which are represented as the sub-components of context. Furthermore, this has been acknowledged by other authors [8] in recognising the significance of 'contexts that are receptive to change' which are pivotal to successful implementation of advanced nursing practice roles within acute and critical care environments. Once again this position is supported in a literature review of international perspectives on advanced nursing practice [18]. In considering the context for implementation of these roles, factors are identified including local conditions, culture of healthcare systems, government policy, nursing needs and healthcare services.

Ireland is one of the few countries in the world that has clearly defined documentation relating to the development of advanced nursing practice and has considered the importance of context in developing a framework with criteria and standards for implementation of these roles. Criteria include responsibilities which cover clinical practice, level of autonomy and expert practice. These are important as previous research [19] undertaken in Canadian acute hospitals, identified that advanced nursing practice roles were developed in response to physician replacement rather than to provide a patient-centred and health-focused service. Advanced nursing roles should enhance the service already being delivered by doctors and not supersede it.

Within the context of advanced nurse practice posts in surgery, that are currently being developed within the NHS (NHS Greater Glasgow and Clyde), it is asserted that these nurses should have the freedom and authority to act autonomously in the assessment, diagnosis, treatment, including prescribing, of patients with multidimensional problems. This includes the authority to refer, admit and discharge within appropriate clinical areas. These roles are integrated within the surgical multidisciplinary team and are focused upon the provision of seamless care, in conjunction with medical staff and other team members. The roles comprise a number of key areas:

- Comprehensive History Taking: The advanced nurse practitioner undertakes comprehensive person-centred assessments of the person's physical, mental, psychological and social needs, strengths and assets—actively involving the person, their families and carers, and wider partners.
- Clinical Assessment: The advanced nurse practitioner undertakes a comprehensive clinical examination of the patient in their entirety, inclusive of: physical examination of all systems, mental health assessment and remote assessment where appropriate.
- Investigations: The advanced nurse practitioner has the freedom and authority to request, where indicated using judgement and clinical reasoning, appropriate diagnostic tests/investigations based on differential diagnoses and interpret/evaluate and analyse previously requested results of tests/investigations working collaboratively with other healthcare professionals when needed.
- Treatment: The advanced nurse practitioner formulates an action plan for the treatment of the patient, synthesising clinical information based on the patient's presentation, history, clinical assessment and findings from relevant investigations, using appropriate evidence-based practice. The advanced nurse practitioner is an independent prescriber and also implements non-pharmacological related interventions/therapies, dependent on situation and technical requirements of care.
- Admission, Discharge and Referral: The advanced nurse practitioner has the freedom and authority to admit and discharge from clinical areas, dependent on patient need at time of review. This includes the freedom and authority to refer to all appropriate health and social care professional groups and agencies, working collaboratively with them.

9.5   Conclusion

In conclusion, nurses play pivotal roles in the provision of emergency general surgery care. The evidence of efficacy of advanced practice nurses, presented in this chapter, correlates closely with a range of international studies [20–23]. Furthermore, it has been clearly demonstrated that advanced practice nurses, undertaking duties traditionally performed by junior doctors in acute hospital settings, can have a positive impact across a range of measures relating to patients, staff and organisational outcomes.

However, the levels of training and education that these nurses have engaged in have been previously emphasised [15] and this is relevant to both autonomous clinical decision-making and the outcomes delivered. This is achieved by engaging in a process of gaining competency [24] through experience, expert knowledge, education and training, and arrived at through consultation with the evidence and considering patient preferences.

In respect of surgical care, it is accepted that advanced practice nurses have the potential to enhance the capability of surgical teams. This, however, will necessitate commitment and active partnership between managers, surgeons, nurses and other surgical staff. It will accordingly provide nurses with a purposeful career path in emergency surgical care and this should be advanced as an approach for working closely with surgeons, having a shared ambition and coherent direction to provide patients with an improved, timely and high quality emergency surgery service.

References

1. Aggarwal G, Peden CJ, Mohammed MA, et al. Evaluation of the collaborative use of an evidence-based care bundle in emergency laparotomy. JAMA Surg. 2019;154(5):e190145. https://doi.org/10.1001/jamasurg.2019.0145.
2. Scott JW, Olufajo OA, Brat GA, et al. Use of national burden to define operative emergency general surgery. JAMA Surg. 2016;151(6):e160480. https://doi.org/10.1001/jamasurg.2016.0480.
3. Coyne I, Comiskey C, Lalor J, Higgins A, Elliot N, Begley C. An exploration of clinical practice in sites with and without clinical nurse or midwife specialists or advanced nurse practitioners, in Ireland. BMC Health Serv Res. 2016;16:151.
4. National Council for the Professional Development of Nursing and Midwifery (NCNM). A preliminary evaluation of the role of the advanced nurse practitioner. Dublin: NCNM; 2005.
5. Dowling M, Beauchesne M, Farrelly F, Murphy K. Int J Nurs Pract. 2013;19(2):131–40. https://doi.org/10.1111/ijn.12050.
6. Watson R, Crump H, Imison C, Currie C, Gaskins M. Emergency general surgery: challenges and opportunities. Research report. London: Nuffield Trust; 2016.
7. Royal College of Surgeons in Ireland (RCSI). Model of care for acute surgery and the national policy and procedure for safe surgery. Royal College of Surgeons in Ireland. 2013. http://www.rcsi.ie/files/surgery/docs/20131030121710_RCSI_Model_of_Care_for_Acute_S.pdf.

8. Woo BFY, Lee JXY, Tam WWS. The impact of the advanced practice nursing role on quality of care, clinical outcomes, patient satisfaction, and cost in the emergency and critical care settings: a systematic review. Hum Resour Health. 2017;15:63.
9. Comiskey C, Coyne I, Lalor J, Begley C. A national cross-sectional study measuring predictors for improved service user outcomes across clinical nurse or midwife specialist, advanced nurse practitioner and control sites. J Adv Nurs. 2014;70(5):1128–37. https://doi.org/10.1111/jan.12273.
10. Swan M, Ferguson S, Chang A, Larson E, Smaldone A. Quality of primary care by advanced practice nurses: a systematic review. Int J Qual Health Care. 2015;27(5):396–404. https://doi.org/10.1093/intqhc/mzv054.
11. Martínez-González NA, Djalali S, Tandjung R, Huber-Geismann F, Markun S, Wensing M, et al. Substitution of physicians by nurses in primary care: a systematic review and meta-analysis. BMC Health Serv Res. 2014;14:214. https://doi.org/10.1186/1472-6963-14-214.
12. Hiza EA, Gottschalk MB, Umpierrez E, Bush P, Reisman WM. Effect of a dedicated orthopaedic advanced practice provider in a level I trauma center: analysis of length of stay and cost. J Orthop Trauma. 2015;29(7):e225–30. https://doi.org/10.1097/BOT.0000000000000261.
13. Morris DS, Reilly P, Rohrbach J, Telford G, Kim P, Sims CA. The influence of unit-based nurse practitioners on hospital outcomes and readmission rates for patients with trauma. J Trauma Acute Care Surg. 2012;73(2):474–8. https://doi.org/10.1097/TA.0b013e31825882bb.
14. Jennings N, Clifford S, Fox AR, O'Connell J, Gardner G. The impact of nurse practitioner services on cost, quality of care, satisfaction and waiting times in the emergency department: a systematic review. Int J Nurs Stud. 2015;52(1):421–35.
15. McDonnell A, Goodwin E, Kennedy FR, et al. An evaluation of the implementation of Advanced Nurse Practitioner (ANP) roles in an acute hospital setting. J Adv Nurs. 2015;71(4):789–99. https://doi.org/10.1111/jan.12558.
16. Stephenson J. Nurses are developing new roles to improve care of laparotomy patients. Nursing Times. 2019. https://www.nursingtimes.net/news/research-and-innovation/nurses-developing-new-roles-to-improve-laparotomy-care/7028566.article
17. McCormack B, Kitson A, Harvey G, Rycroft-Malone J, Titchen A, Seers K. Getting evidence into practice: the meaning of context. J Adv Nurs. 2002;38:94–104.
18. Carney M. International perspectives on advanced nurse and midwife practice, regarding advanced practice, criteria for posts and persons and requirements for regulation of advanced nurse /midwife practice. Blackrock: NMBI; 2016.
19. Dunn K, Nicklin W. The status of advanced nursing roles in Canadian teaching hospitals. Can J Nurs Adm. 1995;8:111–35.
20. Bryant-Lukosius D, Carter N, Reid K, Donald F, Martin-Misener R, Kilpatrick K, et al. The effectiveness and cost effectiveness of clinical nurse specialist-led hospital to home transitional care: a systematic review. J Evaluat Clin Pract. 2015;21(5):763–81. https://doi.org/10.1111/jep.12401.
21. Donald F, Kilpatrick K, Carter N, Bryant-Lukosius D, Martin-Misener R, Kaasalainen S, et al. Hospital to community transitional care by nurse practitioners: a systematic review of cost-effectiveness. Int J Nurs Stud. 2015;52(1):436–51.
22. Newhouse RP, Stanik-Hutt J, White KM, Johantgen M, Bass EB, Zangaro G, et al. Advanced practice nurse outcomes 1990–2008: a systematic review. Nurs Econ. 2011;29(5):1–22.
23. Begley C, Murphy K, Higgins A, Elliott N, Lalor J, Sheerin F, et al. An evaluation of Specialist Clinical Nurse and Midwife Specialist and Advanced Nurse and Midwife Practitioner Roles in Ireland (SCAPE). Dublin: National Council for the Professional Development of Nursing and Midwifery in Ireland; 2010.
24. McConkey RW, Hahessy S. Developing the advanced nursing practice role in non-muscle invasive bladder cancer surveillance in Ireland. Int J Urol Nurs. 2018;12(2–3):91–5.

Data, Registry, Quality Improvement and Patient Outcome Measures

10

Sam Huddart

10.1 Quality Improvement

Batalden and Davidoff defined quality improvement in healthcare as "the combined efforts of everyone—healthcare professionals, patients and their families, researchers, payers, planners and educators—to make the changes that will lead to better patient outcomes (health), better system performance (care) and better professional development (learning)" (Batalden and Davidoff [1]).

Deming WE (1900–1993) is considered by many to be the father of quality improvement science. He is credited with transforming quality in industrial manufacturing in the USA during World War II, in post-war Japan, and at the Ford Motor company in the 1980s. He adapted statistical control methods originally developed by Walter Shewhart (a statistician at Bell laboratories). Shewhart developed control charts that allowed the monitoring of a system and identified common- and special-cause variation. Deming developed a theory of "profound knowledge". For profound knowledge of a particular system we must have: an appreciation of the system; knowledge of the variation within that system; a theory of knowledge (including its concepts and limitations) and knowledge of psychology. Deming theorised that profound knowledge is a pre-requisite to improvement within a system. He also described the PDSA cycle (plan, do, study, act), a cornerstone of Quality Improvement methodology, which is described below.

Quality in healthcare is not a new concept. Avedis Donabedian described the evaluation of quality in medical healthcare [2]. He described quality in healthcare in terms of three distinct domains: structure, process and outcome. Outcome measures are often the mainstay of assessing the quality of a healthcare service. Donabedian

S. Huddart (✉)
Royal Surrey County Hospital, Guildford, UK

SPACeR (Surrey Peri-operative, Anaesthesia & Critical Care Research Group), Guildford, UK
e-mail: samhuddart@nhs.net

© World Society of Emergency Surgery and Donegal Clinical and Research Academy 2020   71
M. Sugrue et al. (eds.), *Resources for Optimal Care of Emergency Surgery*,
Hot Topics in Acute Care Surgery and Trauma,
https://doi.org/10.1007/978-3-030-49363-9_10

discussed the necessity and limitations of outcome measures as an evaluation of quality. Some outcome measures (e.g. mortality) are concrete, unambiguous and relatively easy to measure, others (e.g. patient-reported outcomes or morbidity) are less well-defined. Outcomes give an aggregate assessment of a hospital performance in a given area. However, they lack specificity for the quality of underlying care, do not give an assessment of the processes of care, nor the underlying health-care structures that lead to the outcomes. For example, all high-risk emergency surgical cases are at risk of adverse outcomes (morbidity or mortality). Therefore, the rate of adverse outcome alone cannot be used as a measure of the quality of care in an institution. To assess quality of care key processes must be identified. Compliance to key care measures must be studied alongside outcome measures.

Examining the process and structure-drivers of a particular outcome is a useful method in identifying areas for improvement. This approach allows the construction of driver diagrams that define the primary and secondary drivers of the desired outcome, thereby providing a structure for focusing on areas for quality improvement. An example of a driver diagram is shown in Fig. 10.1.

Biomedical scientific research is essential to further knowledge and understanding, and to focus the development of new treatments and interventions. This answers the question of *why* we should focus clinical trials on a specific subject. This is ideally suited to the gold-standard randomised control trial.

Clinical scientific research is essential to answer the question of *what* the best evidence-based treatment in the clinical setting is (i.e. translation of biomedical research into the clinical setting). Again, this is ideally suited to the gold-standard randomised control trial.

However, there can be a long delay between realisation of new knowledge, and thus identification of best-care, and implementation of that care. One often-quoted

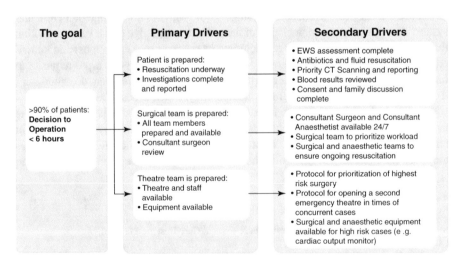

Fig. 10.1 Example of a driver diagram for improving time between the decision for operation to arrival in the operating theatre for emergency surgical patients (EWS—Early Warning Score)

study reports a 17-year delay between new knowledge and widespread implementation [3]. This delay exemplifies the importance of quality improvement systems to implement evidence-based practice and improve care.

Quality improvement science answers the question of *how* best evidence is translated and implemented to the benefit of all patients and not just those in research centres. In other words, it is already established why and what we need to do, what is now needed is a method of reliably translating that knowledge into improving the health of patients in real-world day-to-day medicine.

A review of quality improvement methodology and its use in Intensive Care concluded that "Quality improvement methodology and application does not threaten evidence-based medicine, indeed quality improvement is about the reliable, safe, effective, efficient and timely delivery of the best evidence-based treatment for a patient" [4].

10.2   The Model for Change

The PDSA cycle was originally described by Shewhart in 1931 [5] and further developed by Deming. The PDSA cycle has subsequently been described and recommended for use in the healthcare setting (Fig. 10.2; [6–8]). The four stages are:

Plan	Plan the change to be tested or implemented.
Do	Carry out the test or change.
Study	Studying the data before and after the change and reflect on what was learned.
Act	Plan the next change cycle or full implementation based on what has been learned.

Fig. 10.2 The plan do study act cycle

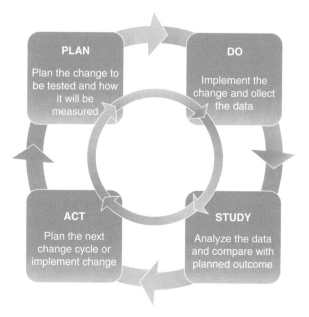

PLAN

Plan the change to be tested and how it will be measured

DO

Implement the change and ollect the data

ACT

Plan the next change cycle or implement change

STUDY

Analyze the data and compare with planned outcome

The model for improvement [7] adds further questions to the PDSA cycle:

1. What are we trying to accomplish?
2. How will we know that a change is an improvement?
3. What changes can we make that will result in an improvement?

The model for improvement has been adopted by international healthcare improvement programmes and organisations (e.g. Surviving Sepsis Campaign, Institute for Healthcare Improvement (USA), Health Foundation (UK), NHS Institute for Innovation and Improvement (UK) and the Kings Fund).

10.3   Measurement of Change

To execute the PDSA cycle we must measure processes. This in itself is a significant challenge and can create resistance to improvement initiatives. Solberg et al. [9] describe three faces of measurement: improvement, accountability and research. Measuring performance in healthcare for accountability and league tables can lead to secular improvement; however, it can lead some clinicians to be resistant to measurement, change and thus improvement. Therefore, in order for measurement to be successful in quality improvement it must focus on improvement and not accountability.

Measurement in improving quality in healthcare should include outcomes and the structure and processes leading to those outcomes [2]. Measurement should also include balancing measures to assess unintended consequences and associated losses [4].

10.4   Examples of Data Registries and Quality Improvement

Publication of process and outcome data has been used effectively in several clinical settings. In the wake of the UK Bristol Heart Enquiry, significant national efforts have been made to improve outcomes after cardiac surgery. In 2001, the public enquiry into outcomes after cardiac surgery at the Bristol Royal Infirmary prompted publication of surgeon-specific outcomes. A 2007 study of 25,730 cardiac procedures demonstrated that mortality after publication of surgeon-specific outcomes was less than before publication (2.4% vs 1.8%, $p = 0.014$), despite an increase in the proportion of high-risk cases after publication of outcomes [10]. In a more recent publication of national data, mortality after coronary artery bypass grafting had reduced by 25% between 2001 and 2008 [11]. Publication of outcomes provides transparency and comparability of care between centres and individuals. This has focused clinicians on their patients' clinical processes and created a culture of continual improvement.

In contrast to emergency general surgery, cardiac surgery is predominantly elective, with little resultant hand-over between surgeons, and a relatively homogenous population of a handful of procedures. Many conditions that result in the need for emergency general surgery develop over time, with various pathways of presentation. Surgeon-specific data in the emergency setting is fraught with the problems of which surgeon to record for which outcome—the admitting surgeon or the operating surgeon. Neither can be held solely responsible for the patients' outcome if they have not been responsible for the entire care of the patient throughout their hospital stay. This is often not the case with on-call patterns. Therefore, unit-specific outcomes would appear to be a better comparable measure of care in emergency general surgery.

In emergency orthopaedic surgery for fractured neck of femur (NOF) in the UK, compulsory data collection and publication of unit-specific data has been launched [12]. The UK National Hip Fracture Database is a joint result of collaborative work between orthopaedic surgeons, anaesthetists and geriatricians. Data collection has led to some units reporting a reduction in mortality and length of hospital stay [13]. Patients presenting with hip fracture share similarities with patients presenting for emergency general surgery, for example they are often elderly with multiple comorbidities. The National Hip Fracture Database is a good example of groups of clinicians coming together to agree best practice and then ensuring widespread implementation.

In the USA, the *American College of Surgeons National Surgical Quality Improvement Program (ACS NSQIP)* has been collecting data from Veterans Health Administration (VHA) hospitals and other hospitals who have subsequently joined the program, since 1994. The ACS NSQIP provides participating hospitals with tools, analysis, reports and guidelines to make informed decisions about improving quality of care. There have been a number of publications demonstrating improvements in mortality, morbidity and hospital length of stay in hospitals after participating in the ACS NSQIP.

The program collects 135 variables including pre-operative risk factors, intraoperative variables, 30-day mortality and morbidity outcomes after surgery. This has led to a complex and comprehensive risk calculator which includes both elective and emergency surgeries, including emergency general surgery procedures. The risk calculator is freely available online. The ACS NSQIP risk calculator has been developed from data from a specific group of hospitals within the US healthcare system. This should be borne in mind when using the calculator to inform risk for patients outside of this healthcare system.

In the UK, there have been a number of programmes developed focusing on high-risk emergency general surgery, namely emergency laparotomy. The culmination of these projects has resulted in the National Emergency Laparotomy Audit (NELA). This is a compulsory national audit and every hospital in England and Wales is duty-bound to submit data on all general-surgical patients undergoing non-elective major abdominal surgery. Patient data collection started in December 2013 and will continue to December 2020 and potentially beyond. Alongside patient data (process and outcome), NELA has also organisational data (structure). NELA publish national and hospital-level data to aid quality improvement and have developed a risk prediction tool specifically for NELA inclusive patients.

10.5   Data

Accurate data collection, processing and dissemination is key to monitoring and improving processes and patient outcomes. The use of national data registries allows benchmarking of performance of individual centres against the average, best and worst practice of other centres. In addition, it allows setting of targets that can be used as a measure of the quality of care at individual institutions. Publication of this data informs patient choice and funding, as well as inspiring best practice.

10.5.1 Structure Measures

Healthcare structure impacts on patient care. Numbers and levels of hospital beds per population, staffing level and access to facilities (e.g. emergency theatre, intensive care, urgent imaging) all contribute to a healthcare centre's ability to deliver high quality care to their patients and maximise the likelihood of favourable outcome. Data registries should include measures to demonstrate and benchmark access to care and facilities within an individual institution.

10.5.2 Process Measures

Data collection should include key process measures of patient care. There is no agreed standard of minimum data set for monitoring compliance to patient care process measures and will depend on the setting of the healthcare system. There are advantages to large, complex and detailed data sets including potentially increased validity and specificity of risk prediction models calculated from the data. However, large detailed data sets provide additional resource implications to ensure that data is collected and is accurate. There is therefore a compromise between detail of data sets and ease of collection. Several established data sets collect detailed data yet routinely report only key process measures. For example, the National Emergency Laparotomy Audit in the UK collects detailed patient-level data. However, the yearly national reports and quarterly hospital reports detail only key metrics. The collection of additional data above these simplified metrics is necessary to allow more detailed investigation should a centre have measures that are above or below the accepted range of expected performance.

10.5.3 Outcome Measures

Outcome measures are essential to assessing the product of healthcare provision. Ideally, they should include morbidity, mortality (short vs long), unanticipated return to operating theatre, unanticipated admission to intensive care, destination on discharge and patient-reported outcome measures (PROMs).

There are a number of measures of morbidity after surgery described in the literature. There is no consensus as to the best measures. It is important that, within a QI data set, the same measures are used in order to allow valid comparison of outcomes between centres. Examples include the Clavien–Dindo classification and the Post-Operative Morbidity Survey (POMS). The NSQIP database uses its own definitions of morbidity. The National Emergency Laparotomy Audit does not include morbidity measures beyond return to theatre and unanticipated intensive care admission.

In the emergency setting, mortality is dependent on underlying acute pathology, and physiological response to acute illness and underlying comorbidities. Presentation and severity of surgical emergencies are sporadic, therefore mortality from them will also vary over time. This variation should be accounted for when comparing outcomes at different centres. Data collection should include routine collection of data to predict the risk of mortality. This can be used to risk-adjust mortality outcomes, thereby accounting for variations in severity of illness presenting to different centres and over time. In addition, predicted mortality can be used as an adjunct for individual patient consent and decision-making.

10.5.4 Collaboration

Benchmarking structure, process and outcome measures against other hospitals is a powerful means of driving improvement. It also allows identification of hospitals with excellent performance data and should inspire other hospitals to collaborate and improve.

10.6   Risk Prediction

Mortality and morbidity risk prediction can be used to inform patients and their relatives, to prompt escalation in care for high-risk patients and to adjust observed outcomes for risk. There are a number of validated tools for risk prediction in the emergency surgical patients. In the USA, the recommended tool is the NSQUIP risk calculator (http://riskcalculator.facs.org/RiskCalculator/). In the UK, the National Emergency Laparotomy Audit (NELA) has used data from over 20,000 emergency major abdominal general surgery cases to recalibrate existing risk prediction models. The NELA risk prediction tool is specific for emergency major general surgery [14].

10.6.1 Examples of Quality Improvement in Emergency Surgery

In the UK, the Emergency Laparotomy network collected data on consecutive emergency major general surgery patients over a 3-month period from 35 NHS hospitals. They observed a crude mortality of 14.6%, with mortality rates varying widely between centres [15]. From this, the National Emergency Laparotomy Audit was developed. This compulsory national audit collects data from all acute hospitals in England and Wales. This substantial audit collected over 20,000 cases in year one (2013–2014), rising to nearly 24,000 in year four (2016–2017). Crude mortality in year one was 11.8% falling to 9.5% in year four (http://nela.org.uk/reports). This apparent improvement will, in part, be due to a multitude of local quality improvement initiatives, some of which has been published in the literature.

The Emergency Laparotomy Pathway Quality Improvement Care (ELPQuiC) bundle used quality improvement methodology to implement a six-step care bundle (early warning scores, sepsis management, consultant led care, early surgical intervention, goal-directed fluid therapy, post-operative intensive care) in four UK NHS hospitals. Using a pre-post cohort design, compliance to the majority of care bundle elements improved in all hospitals. Overall risk-adjusted 30-day mortality was 15.6% before and 9.6% (38% relative reduction) after intervention (95% CI = 0.451–0.836; $p = 0.002$) [16]. In a multicentre study, Moller et al. implemented a multimodal, multidisciplinary care protocol for patients with peptic ulcer perforation. Mortality was 27% for control groups and 17.1% for intervention group ($p = 0.005$) and relative risk of 0.63 (95% CI = 0.41–0.97), a relative risk reduction of 37 (5–58) per cent and a number needed to treat of 10 (6–38) [17].

The Emergency Laparotomy Collaborative (ELC) project implemented a six-point care bundle similar to that used in the ELPQuiC project [18]. The bundle included prompt measurement of blood lactate levels, early sepsis assessment and treatment, transfer to the operating room within defined time goals after the decision to operate, use of goal-directed fluid therapy, post-operative admission to an intensive care unit, and multidisciplinary involvement of senior clinicians in the decision and delivery of perioperative care. The project was implemented across 28 UK National Health Service Hospitals simultaneously in all hospitals (October 2015 to September 2017). Regular quality improvement and leadership training was provided during collaborative meetings of ELC teams throughout the project. Risk-adjusted mortality fell from 5.3% pre-ELC to 4.5% in the second year of the project. Mean length of stay was reduced by 1.2 days over the course of implementation. These improvements in outcome were associated with improvements in compliance with five out of six of the bundle elements [18]. However, the trial was designed as a quality improvement project and as such cannot infer any causal relationships between observed improvements in process measures and outcomes.

The Enhanced Peri-Operative Care for High-risk Patients (EPOCH) trial was a step-wedge randomised control design across 93 UK NHS hospitals. During the intervention, a 37-component care intervention was implemented for all patients undergoing emergency major general surgery, utilising the NELA database. Hospitals were randomised to introduce the quality improvement care pathway at various times over the 85-week trial period. The treatment period was between March 2014 and October 2015. Hospital teams were given QI training prior to implementation. Standard care (pre intervention) patients were compared to patients in the QI group (8484 vs 7374). No difference was observed in primary outcome; 90-day (crude) mortality was 16% for both groups. The study reported only modest changes in process measures despite reportedly good clinician engagement. The authors attributed this to limited time and resources to implement change [19]. This observation may explain the success of other QI initiatives and not the EPOCH trial. Improvements in outcomes observed in the ELPQuiC and ELC projects may be associated with a longer QI period and greater QI resources than that used in EPOCH. In an analysis of the EPOCH QI process, participants reported wide variation in QI and only 11 of 37 process elements were attempted to be improved by more than 50% of participants. Participants also reported significant obstructions to improvement in the time available [20]. Adequate attention must be paid to differences in individual organisations, particularly in relation to cultural differences and willingness to change. Quality improvement programmes require enthusiasm, time and resources in order not only for successful implementation but also to detect improvements.

10.7 Development of Key Performance Indicators

There are a number of key themes that run through the ongoing and published emergency surgery literature. Key performance indicators have been developed from these to address six critical clinical aspects of the care of emergency surgical patients.

1. Data collection, monitoring and system response.
   (a) Data collection is a pre-requisite to any quality monitoring, assurance and imporvement.
2. Early warning score: All emergency surgical patients should have physiological observation data measured at regular intervals appropriate for severity of presenting condition using a track and trigger (early warning) scoring system.
   (a) Early warning track and trigger systems are well established and should be used routinely for all emergency surgery patients with robust escalation protocols [21, 22].
3. Consultant led care.
   (a) There is a paucity of evidence supporting the benefit of seniority of surgical and anaesthetic staff. However, UK national enquires into perioperative death (NCEPOD) have repeatedly reported inappropriately junior surgical and anaesthetic seniority as a potential contributing factor to deaths after surgery. In the UK, patient with a predicted mortality of >5% should have direct consultant led perioperative care [23].
4. Sepsis management.
   (a) Delays in antibiotics and source control have been shown to correlate with worsening mortality in sepsis [24]. The surviving sepsis campaign [25] is well established and compliance to their recommendations should be monitored, improved and maintained.

5. Decision-to-theatre within recommended timing for clinical urgency.
    (a) Once the decision for theatre has been made, emergency surgery should be prioritised according to perceived need and urgency. The UK NCEPOD urgency criteria have been adapted by NELA and are used to monitor compliance to designated time frames:
    - Immediate (1)—within a maximum of 2 h.
    - Urgent (2a)—less than 6 h.
    - Urgent (2b)—less than 18 h.
    - Expedited (3)—at a time convenient for patient and/or clinical team (http://www.nela.org.uk).
6. Post-operative intensive care.
    (a) There is a paucity of evidence for the routine admission of surgical patients to intensive care. There is some evidence demonstrating that hospitals with better access to intensive care (more ICU beds per hospital bed) have significantly better outcomes after surgery [26]. There is also observational evidence that unplanned admissions to intensive care from surgical wards after surgery correlates to a very high mortality risk (39%) [27]. The Royal College of Surgeons of England and the UK Department of Health recommend that patients with a predicted mortality of >10% are cared for in an intensive care setting after high-risk surgery [23]. Subsequent to the publication of these guidelines, the National Emergency Laparotomy Audit has reduced this recommended threshold to 5% (http://www.nela.org.uk).

In addition to these clinical KPIs, there are 5 KPIs for quality improvement (governance and structure), evidence for these are included in the body of the text:

1. Data collection, monitoring and system response.
2. Multidisciplinary teamwork and inter-hospital collaboration.
3. Sequential data analysis and response (PDSA).
4. Institutional management support.
5. Dissemination of learning.

References

1. Batalden P, Davidoff F. What is "quality Improvement" and how can it transform healthcare? Qual Saf Health Care. 2007;16:2–3.
2. Donabedian A. Evaluating the quality of medical care. Milbank Q. 1966;44(3, part 2):166–206.
3. Balas EA, Boren SA. Managing clinical knowledge for health care improvement. In: Bemmel J, AT MC, editors. Yearbook of medical informatics 2000: patient-centered systems. Stuttgart: Schattauer Verlagsgesellschaft mbH; 2000. p. 65–70. http://hdl.handle.net/10675.2/617990. Accessed July 2018.
4. Peden C, Rooney K. The science of improvement as it relates to quality and safety in the ICU. J Intens Care Soc. 2009;10(4):260–5.

5. Shewhart WA. Economic control of quality of manufactured product. New York: D Van Nostrand Company, 1931. (Reprinted by ASQC Quality Press, 1980).
6. Berwick DM. A primer on leading the improvement of systems. BMJ. 1996;312(7031):619–22.
7. Langley G, Nolan K, Nolan T, Norman C, Provost L. The improvement guide: a practical approach to enhancing organizational performance. 2nd ed. San Francisco: Jossey-Bass Publishers; 2009.
8. The Institute for Healthcare Improvement. 2012. http://www.ihi.org/resources/Pages/HowtoImprove/default.aspx. Accessed July 2018.
9. Solberg IL, Mosser G, McDonald S. The three faces of performance measurement: improvement, accountability, and research. Joint Comm J Qual Improv. 1997;23(3):135–47.
10. Bridgewater B, Grayson AD, Brooks N, Grotte G, Fabri BM, Au J, Hooper T, Jones M, Keogh B. Has the publication of cardiac surgery outcome data been associated with changes in practice in northwest England: an analysis of 25,730 patients undergoing CABG surgery under 30 surgeons over eight years. Heart. 2007;93(6):744–8.
11. Bridgewater B, Grant S, Hickey G, Fazal N. National Adult Cardiac Surgery Audit 2010–2011, National Institute for Cardiovascular Outcomes Research (NICOR). 2011. https://www.ucl.ac.uk/nicor/audits/adultcardiac/documents/reports/annualreport2010-11. Accessed July 2018.
12. Currie C, Partridge M, Plant F, Roberts J, Wakeman R, Williams A. The national hip fracture database national report 2012. 2012. http://www.nhfd.co.uk/003/hipfractureR.nsf/0/da44e3a946a14e4180257a6f001eb4db/$FILE/NHFD. National Report 2012.pdf. Accessed July 2018.
13. Gunasekera N, Boulton C, Morris C, Moran C. Hip fracture audit: the Nottingham experience. Osteoporos Int. 2010;21(Suppl 4):S647–53.
14. Eugene N, Oliver CM, Bassett MG, Poulton TE, Kuryba A, Johnston C, Anderson ID, Moonesinghe SR, Grocott MP, Murray DM, Cromwell DA, Walker K, NELA collaboration. Development and internal validation of a novel risk adjustment model for adult patients undergoing emergency laparotomy surgery: the National Emergency Laparotomy Audit risk model. Br J Anaesth. 2018;121(4):739–48.
15. Saunders DI, Murray D, Pichel AC, Varley S, Peden CJ. Variations in mortality after emergency laparotomy: the first report of the UK Emergency Laparotomy Network. Br J Anaesth. 2012;109(3):368–75.
16. Huddart S, Peden CJ, Swart M, McCormick B, Dickinson M, Mohammed MA, Quiney N. Use of a pathway quality improvement care bundle to reduce mortality after emergency laparotomy. Br J Surg. 2015;102(1):57–66.
17. Møller MH, Adamsen S, Thomsen RW, Møller AM, on behalf of the Peptic Ulcer Perforation (PULP) trial group. Multicentre trial of a perioperative protocol to reduce mortality in patients with peptic ulcer perforation. Control Clin Trial. 2011;98(6):802–10.
18. Aggarwal G, Peden CJ, Mohammed MA, Pullyblank A, Williams B, Stephens T, Kellett S, Kirkby-Bott J, Quiney N, Emergency Laparotomy Collaborative. Evaluation of the collaborative use of an evidence-based care bundle in emergency laparotomy. JAMA Surg. 2019;154(5):e190145.
19. Peden CJ, Stephens T, Martin G, Kahan BC, Thomson A, Rivett K, Wells D, Richardson G, Kerry S, Bion J, Pearse RM, Enhanced Peri-Operative Care for High-risk patients (EPOCH) trial group. Effectiveness of a national quality improvement programme to improve survival after emergency abdominal surgery (EPOCH): a stepped-wedge cluster-randomised trial. Lancet. 2019;393(10187):2213–21.
20. Stephens TJ, Peden CJ, Pearse RM, Shaw SE, TEF A, Jones EL, Kocman D, Martin G, EPOCH trial group. Improving care at scale: process evaluation of a multi-component quality improvement intervention to reduce mortality after emergency abdominal surgery (EPOCH trial). Implement Sci. 2018;13(1):142.
21. Hodgetts TJ, Kenward G, Vlachonikolis IG, Payne S, Castle N. The identification of risk factors for cardiac arrest and formulation of activation criteria to alert a medical emergency team. Resuscitation. 2002;54:125–31.

22. National Institute for Health and Clinical Excellence. NICE clinical guideline 50. Acutely ill patients in hospital: National Institute for Health and Clinical Excellence. 2007. http://www.nice.org.uk/CG50. Accessed 30 Jan 2014.
23. Royal College of Surgeons of England, Department of Health. The higher risk general surgical patient: towards improved care for a forgotten group. 2012. http://www.rcseng.ac.uk/publications/docs/higher-risk-surgical-patient/. Accessed 1 Mar 2014.
24. Kumar A, Ellis P, Arabi Y, Roberts D, Light B, Parrillo JE, Dodek P, et al. Initiation of inappropriate antimicrobial therapy results in a fivefold reduction of survival in human septic shock. Chest. 2009;136(5):1237–48.
25. Dellinger RP, Levy MM, Rhodes A, Annane D, Gerlach H, Opal SM et al. Surviving Sepsis Campaign Guidelines Committee including the Pediatric Subgroup. Surviving Sepsis Campaign: international guidelines for management of severe sepsis and septic shock, 2012. Intensive Care Med. 2013;39:165–228.
26. Symons NRA, Moorthy K, Almoudaris AM, Bottle A, Aylin P, Vincent CA. Mortality in high-risk emergency general surgical admissions. Br J Surg. 2013;100:1318–25.
27. Pearse RM, Harrison DA, James P, Watson D, Hinds C, Rhodes A, Grounds RM, Bennett ED. Identification and characterisation of the high-risk surgical population in the United Kingdom. Crit Care. 2006;10(3):R81.

Research in Emergency General Surgery

11

Fausto Catena, Gennaro Perrone, Elena Bonati,
Antonio Tarasconi, Andrew Kirkpatrick, and Ron Maier

11.1 Introduction

The development of units of emergency general surgery (EGS) has confirmed over the years what we already hypothesized is that a dynamic system of emergency surgery, dedicated multidisciplinary teams (surgical, anesthetic, nursing, etc.), trained and competent in EGS, with adequate resources, both in terms of the availability of these people and of institutional resources to provide assistance, have led to a marked improvement in the results in this field [1].

This discipline, even if not codified, has always been at the basis of personal care and the provision of necessary care that every hospital must guarantee. Nevertheless only recently has it been recognized and promoted as a holistic body of dedicated surgical practice, worthy of study and organization. Even today many metrics relating to this discipline remain scarcely researched and controversial. The collected data showed that devoting resources and giving priority to the EGS service improved the results. Hospitals with dedicated EGS services seem to have reduced operating times and leaner protocols for common EGS procedures that lead to faster and more effective treatment [2].

F. Catena · G. Perrone (✉) · A. Tarasconi
Department of Emergency Surgery, Maggiore Hospital, Parma, Italy

E. Bonati
General Surgical Clinic, Maggiore Hospital, Parma, Italy

A. Kirkpatrick
HBI, Department of Medicine, The University of Calgary, Calgary, AB, Canada
e-mail: andrew.kirkpatrick@albertahealthservices.ca

R. Maier
Harborview Medical Center, Seattle, WA, USA
e-mail: ronmaier@uw.edu

© World Society of Emergency Surgery and Donegal Clinical and Research Academy 2020   83
M. Sugrue et al. (eds.), *Resources for Optimal Care of Emergency Surgery*,
Hot Topics in Acute Care Surgery and Trauma,
https://doi.org/10.1007/978-3-030-49363-9_11

The EGS model provides a safe surgical environment for patients and is associated with a reduced complication rate for the most widespread interventions in these units such as appendectomy and laparoscopic cholecystectomy for acute cholecystitis. Overall, the EGS model translated into better results for patients with acute general surgery conditions [3].

Many questions related to critical elements such as efficiency, cost-effectiveness, and value still not answered today. Patients undergoing general urgent surgery treated at the trauma centers incurred higher costs than those treated in other facilities, regardless of patient severity. These costs almost doubled for those admitted to intensive care units. Given the recent increase in EGS, further investigations are needed to better understand the reasons for this cost differential [4].

The implementation and development of research on EGS services will benefit patients and professional satisfaction of the surgeon. Ultimately, the research must understand whether the EGS service models provide better results for sick patients in need of urgent surgery. Therefore, high-level data is needed to answer these fundamental questions and guide initiatives for continuous quality improvement. Answer all questions related to any category of illness, procedure, model of assistance, etc. requires accurate and complete data.

Some studies such as Murphy have exploited Donebian's less recent study which already in 1988 has extrapolated a structure model for EGS with the aim of making best use of both the structure and the perspectives of several stakeholders [5, 6].

Already in 2016 the working group led by F Catena, M Sugrue, R Maier, and AW Kirkpatrick was responsible for writing a chapter in the manual entitled Resources for Care of Acute Surgery, which introduced the Key Performance Indicators (KPI) of primary level and highest level for an academic EGS. This work was an initial demonstration of Institutional Commitment to Research in EGS. Research on modeling EGS services from jobs like this will surely benefit. The effort of the aforementioned group to generate a set of simple but generalizable key KPIs was the first input to institutions in fostering research in this field. The greatest difficulties have emerged in identifying appropriate measurable criteria or metrics that can reflect quality or even quality potential through the countless healthcare and provider systems that attempt this service. This foundation from the Donegal Summit is hoping to generate potential KPIs which can be both debated by leaders in EGS Research and thereafter subjected to prospective validation through patient and provider outcomes. Therefore the KPIs are used to examine and eventually evaluate the potential of an institution's research structure, the method of conducting research and, finally, whether the Institution will be able to translate the energy used in research with valid studies that can potentially guide and improve patient care worldwide.

11.2 Can the Emergency Surgeon Be a Researcher?

A review of all the published articles related to the research methodology in EGS and collection of information from companies, universities, and governmental organizations was performed to create a menu of existing methodological research specifically related to EGS. These principles have been explained with putative KPIs that have been the basis of the debate among experts in the field.

As widely demonstrated by recent studies, the EGS research KPIs are very important for emergency surgery. A healthy academic environment is necessary for an effective EGS service as a well-established research activity is the engine of effective continuous medical education.

The permanent medical education, if effective, and its association with initiatives of continuous quality improvement are the basis of the highest standard clinical activity that guarantees high-level clinical performance [7–12].

It is essential to consider the KPIs describing all the retrospective performance and results, prospective Level 1 Evidence Based Medicine (EBM) activities and tangible indicators of research output.

For this reason the first KPI was the maintenance of a database/clinical registry (retrospective/prospective) in order to have updated documentation of clinical activity together with the ability to extract data to perform all or some of the retrospective analysis with univariate/multivariate evaluations and correspondence of the propensity score. The "evidence based" limit of this type of research is clear but these studies constitute the basis for identifying possible prospective trials and for an effective planning of randomized controlled trials. There is also a formal requirement for regular audits of data quality/accuracy for this clinical database/registry. Having an updated database annually allows you to enter at least 90% of patients who access the EGS obtaining a ratio between accesses to the service/insertions in the database almost optimal.

The second KPI focuses on demonstrating the institutional capacity to organize at least one randomized controlled study every 5 years. For our group, both for experienced and reported experiences, this is a very challenging KPI, but considering the importance of generating Level 1-based research in the field of surgery, this requirement is fundamental. Randomized controlled trials are still limited in surgical research, but they remain the main engines of excellence in clinical science.

Less than 10% of the clinical studies reported in the surgical journals are RCTs, and the surgical trials reach a percentage of 50% of RCT compared to those of internal medicine. EGS centers will be needed to invest resources on this type of research with the production of at least one RCT every 5 years. It is important to underline that it must be a single-center RCT or alternatively a multicentric RCT with a primary role in making its contribution.

The assignment of a modest numerical threshold is due to the immense commitment in terms of protocol writing, approval of the ethics committee, clinical initiation, conduct, analysis, and publication for an investigator-sponsored non-industry supported RCT. It is duly noted that multicentre RCTs compound these challenges greatly.

The last three KPIs reflect tangible measure of scientific production/activity. These reflect thresholds of five full articles in indexed journals per year, international and national scientific presentations, and committed research activity of trainees, the most valuable resource for future academic capital.

Moreover, at least one paper must be in medium-high impact factors journals (>1.0). Since there is no standard evaluation of the quality of scientific congress presentations, only complete articles in indexed journals and not abstract books should be the best choice.There is a minimum requested standard to publish a full article on indexed journals. Although ambitious, this threshold for the objectives of published manuscripts does not seem to be too high in our view; reflecting on the current possibility of publishing complete articles has greatly increased by the huge number of indexed journals and by the opportunities for quick online publication. Thus in a high-level emergency surgery center with a well-organized clinical database it should not be unreasonable to find research fellows along with attendings and residents that are able to direct scientific projects that result in five full paper publications in indexed journals even if there are a limited number of staff.

11.3 Conclusions

This document obtained from the Donegal summit outlines a minimum standard for the future and establishes the reference points of research on EGS and measurable KPIs. An active research program at national, regional, and institutional level in EGS will optimize service delivery, identify gaps, and improve security and outcome. The KPIs emerging in this document are a beginning for this process.

References

1. Murphy PB, Paskar D, Hilsden R, Koichopolos J, Mele TS, on behalf of Western Ontario Research Collaborative on Acute Care Surgery. Acute care surgery: a means for providing cost-effective, quality care for gallstone pancreatitis. World J Emerg Surg. 2017;12:20.
2. Cubas RF, Gómez NR, Rodriguez S, Wanis M, Sivanandam A, Garberoglio CA. Outcomes in the management of appendicitis and cholecystitis in the setting of a new acute care surgery service model: impact on timing and cost. J Am Coll Surg. 2012;215(5):715–21. https://doi.org/10.1016/j.jamcollsurg.2012.06.415.
3. Nagaraja V, Eslick GD, Cox MR. The acute surgical unit model verses the traditional "on call" model: a systematic review and meta-analysis. World J Surg. 2014;38(6):1381–7. https://doi.org/10.1007/s00268-013-2447-1.
4. Narayan M, Tesoriero R, Bruns BR, Klyushnenkova EN, Chen H, Diaz JJ. Acute care surgery: defining the economic burden of emergency general surgery. J Am Coll Surg. 2016;222(4):691–9. https://doi.org/10.1016/j.jamcollsurg.2016.01.054.
5. Murphy PB, Vogt KN, Mele TS, Hameed SM, Ball CG, Parry NG. Timely surgical care for acute biliary disease: an indication of quality. Ann Surg. 2016;264(6):913–4.
6. Donabedian A. The quality of care. How can it be assessed? JAMA. 1988;260:1743–8.
7. Kluger Y, Catena F, Kashuk J, Ansaloni L. World Society of Emergency Surgery—indication of globalism and renaissance through the 2015 biennial assembly. World J Emerg Surg. 2015;10:40.
8. Catena F, Moore F, Ansaloni L, Leppäniemi A, Sartelli M, Peitzmann AB, et al. Emergency surgeon: "last of the mohicans" 2014–2016 editorial policy WSES-WJES:position papers, guidelines, courses, books and original research; from WJES impact factor to WSES congress impact factor. World J Emerg Surg. 2014;9(1):25.

9. MacLehose RR, Reeves BC, Harvey IM, Sheldon TA, Russell IT, Black AM. A systematic review of comparisons of effect sizes derived from randomised and non-randomised studies. Health Technol Assess. 2000;4(34):1–154.

10. Arkenbosch J, Miyagaki H, Kumara HM, Yan X, Cekic V, Whelan RL. Efficacy of laparoscopic-assisted approach for reversal of Hartmann's procedure: results from the American College of Surgeons National Surgical Quality Improvement Program (ACS-NSQIP) database. Surg Endosc. 2015;29(8):2109–14.

11. Chana P, Burns EM, Arora S, Darzi AW, Faiz OD. A systematic review of theimpact of dedicated emergency surgical services on patient outcomes. Ann Surg. 2016;263(1):20–7.

12. Kao LS, Tyson JE, Blakely ML, Lally KP. Clinical research methodology I: introduction to randomized trials. J Am Coll Surg. 2008;206(2):361–9.

Position Paper on Education and Training in Emergency Surgery

12

Michael Sugrue, Mark W. Bowyer, Leo Lawler, Isidro Martinez, and Lyndsay Pearce

Quality outcomes in emergency surgery require a dynamic efficient emergency surgery system, coupled with surgical teams trained and competent in Acute Care Surgery. Education with known competencies must encompass interaction across all disciplines [1–3]. Given the burden of emergency surgery in medicine globally and the opportunity to improve care this paper will outline a vision for Education and Training in Emergency Surgery.

The aim of this chapter is to outline key standards and develop measurement KPIs. This foundation from the Donegal 2016 Summit on Emergency Surgery will lead to a future where these can be validated with patient and provider outcomes.

M. Sugrue (✉)
Letterkenny University Hospital and University Hospital Galway,
Letterkenny, Donegal, Ireland

EU INTERREG Emergency Surgery Outcomes Advancement Project (eSOAP),
Letterkenny University Hospital, Letterkenny, Donegal, Ireland

M. W. Bowyer
The Department of Surgery, Uniformed Services University
and Walter Reed National Military Medical Center, Bethesda, MD, USA
e-mail: mark.bowyer@usuhs.edu

L. Lawler
Mater Misericordiae University Hospital, Dublin, Ireland
e-mail: llawler@mater.ie

I. Martinez
HFEBS EmSurg, Servicio de Cirugía General y Digestiva,
Complejo Hospitalario de Jaén, Jaén, Spain

L. Pearce
Salford Royal Hospital, Salford, UK
e-mail: Lyndsay.pearce@srft.nhs.uk

© World Society of Emergency Surgery and Donegal Clinical and Research Academy 2020   89
M. Sugrue et al. (eds.), *Resources for Optimal Care of Emergency Surgery*,
Hot Topics in Acute Care Surgery and Trauma,
https://doi.org/10.1007/978-3-030-49363-9_12

Table 12.1 Key standards in education in emergency surgery care	Expectation for education culture and environment
	Governance and resource management
	Facilitating learners
	Supporting surgical educators
	Supporting multidisciplinary team work approach
	Curricula development accreditation and performance assessment
	Innovation and skills development
	Access to learning opportunities in emergency surgery
	Accreditation of education and competency assessment

12.1 Methods

This chapter reviews all published articles relating to Education and Training in Emergency Surgery and collation of information from learned societies, colleges and government organizations to create a menu of existing education courses and platforms. These KPI's will deal with both under- and postgraduate education in emergency surgery, the interaction across different disciplines and communities. The overarching philosophies from education in emergency surgery care are shown in Table 12.1. Each of these key standards will have a KPI developed.

12.2 Results

Well-defined, standards and guidelines in emergency surgery education do not exist, despite some significant recent publications and improved implementation of training [4–7]. Acute care receiving hospitals need to accept and implement education systems which are documented and validated. Nationally agreed validation and accreditation of educational curricula should be a requirement of all acute surgical care units and in undergraduate training.

Postgraduate surgical trainees need to be in practices with embedded acute surgical training competencies. Hospitals receiving emergency surgical patients will need to have a formal visible and documented emergency surgery training programme allocating a minimum of 2 hours per month for trainees education. The hospital will need a Director of Emergency Surgical Training. This position will need resources, time and training facility. The Director of Emergency Surgical Training would be required to write an annual report of educational activities and sign off on completed competencies.

Education activities should engage with other disciplines, particularly Emergency Medicine, Radiology, Gastroenterology and Anaesthesia. This should occur daily as a standard part of workflow and as part of regular case reviews. Where the hospital functions as a referral centre, the referring hospitals will need to be in the education net.

Access to relevant emergency surgery educational materials and resources may surprisingly be difficult. The hospital and system will need documented electronic knowledge transfer mechanisms. This would include email groups, web site linkages and clearly visible emergency surgery course calendars for both educators and trainees.

Chief resident and Senior registrars in the Unit should be encouraged to undertake European Board of Surgery Qualification in Emergency Surgery. This 2-stage quality validation process consists of an eligibility assessment and an examination leading to the award of the title "Fellow of the European Board of Surgery in Emergency Surgery—F.E.B.S./EmSurg".

A UEMS fellowship (F.E.B.S.) would offer a high-level validated quality controlled process reflecting knowledge and skills in emergency surgery.

12.3   Conclusion

This paper outlines a minimal standard for the future options for education in emergency general surgery and suggests some benchmark and measurable KPIs.

Key Performance Education Indicators

Education and training	KPI title	Hospital administration demonstrated support for emergency surgery education
2.	Description	Hospitals receiving emergency surgery patients have a policy and procedure supportive of emergency surgery education, with minimum requirements for not only surgery, but across other disciplines including Emergency Medicine, Radiology, Gastroenterology and Nursing.
3.	Rationale	Without continuous education, focusing on surgical staff, but across main disciplines, patient care will be sub-optimal. Surgical trainees involved in emergency care will need to have documented 1 h/2 weeks in formal emergency surgery education.
4.	Target	One written policy and procedure with measurable education activity for emergency surgery
5.	KPI collection frequency	Semi-annually
6.	KPI reporting frequency	Semi-annually
7.	KPI calculation	Yes/no written policy with verification every 6 months
8.	Reporting aggregation	Hospital
9.	Data source(s)	Hospital administration

Education and training	KPI title	Hospital administration demonstrated support for consultant and trainee teaching of emergency surgery
2.	Description	Hospitals receiving emergency surgery patients have a policy and procedure supportive of the providers of emergency surgery education, to include time allowance with remuneration.
3.	Rationale	Provision of focused education has not been a priority in hospital ethos, falling well behind clinical care and research. Trainees themselves can be involved in education particularly the more senior trainees
4.	Target	Written policy and procedure with documented education activity for emergency surgery teachers, both consultant and trainees.
5.	KPI collection frequency	Semi-annually
6.	KPI reporting frequency	Semi-annually
7.	KPI calculation	Yes/no written policy with verification every 6 months
8.	Reporting aggregation	Hospital
9.	Data source(s)	Hospital administration
Education and training	KPI title	Medical students have a formal attachment to on call surgeons and surgical teams
2.	Description	Medical students education should have dealt with common surgical emergencies. They should have experienced at least two nights on call.
3.	Rationale	Theoretical undergraduate education needs to be reinforced with real clinical situations in order to understand and comprehend acquired knowledge.
4.	Target	90% of students doing a rotation in general surgery should experience at least two certified nights on call
5.	KPI collection frequency	Annually
6.	KPI reporting frequency	Annually
7.	KPI calculation	Annual number of night shifts with certified student presence/ total number of students rotating annually in the service
8.	Reporting aggregation	Hospital 1
9.	Data source(s)	Chair Department of Surgery Director of Surgical Training
Education and training	KPI title	Hospital demonstrate an active electronic-web based continual support for sharing of information in emergency surgery among all groups dealing with emergency surgery patients
2.	Description	Hospitals receiving emergency surgery patients have a policy and procedure identifying electronic networks for dissemination of both existing and new educational information in emergency surgery
3.	Rationale	Creating a learning environment that promotes access to educational material is essential, both to upskill providers and provide immediate answers to clinical care questions

Education and training	KPI title	Hospital demonstrate an active electronic-web based continual support for sharing of information in emergency surgery among all groups dealing with emergency surgery patients
4.	Target	Proven electronic networks sharing educational material in emergency surgery
5.	KPI collection frequency	Semi-annually
6.	KPI reporting frequency	Semi-annually
7.	KPI calculation	Yes/no written policy with verification every 6 months
8.	Reporting aggregation	Hospital
9.	Data source(s)	Chair Department of Surgery
Education and training	KPI title	Ensure attendance at emergency surgery educational course
2.	Description	Hospitals receiving emergency surgery patients mandate that surgical providers of emergency surgery attend a minimum of one CME approved course containing streams that deal with emergency surgery care
3.	Rationale	Well-educated emergency surgery providers ensure the best patient outcomes. Patient safety will be enhanced. In addition, staff satisfaction will increase creating a palpable positive efficient working environment
4.	Target	80% doctors on call attended at CME recognized emergency surgery educational course or general surgery course with an emergency stream
5.	KPI collection frequency	Annually
6.	KPI reporting frequency	Annually
7.	KPI calculation	Numerator divided by denominator expressed as a percentage Numerator: Number of doctors on the emergency on call roster Denominator: Number of doctors on the emergency on call roster who had attended a surgical course
8.	Reporting aggregation	Hospital 1
9.	Data source(s)	Chair Department of Surgery Director of Surgical Training

References

1. Harkin D, Beard J, Wyatt M, Shearman C. Vascular Society UK workforce report. In: Society V, editor. http://www.vascularsociety.org.uk/wp-content/uploads/2014/07/VS-UK-Workforce-Report.pdf. p. 25.
2. Garrett K, Kaups KL. The aging surgeon: when is it time to leave active practice? Bull Am Coll Surg. 2014;99(4):32–5.
3. Greenaway D. Securing the future of excellent patient care. The Shape of Training. http://www.shapeoftraining.co.uk/static/documents/content/Shape_of_training_FINAL_Report.pdf_53977887.pdf.

4. Ferguson H, Fitzgerald E, Shalhoub J, Gokani V, Beamish A. The shape of training review 2013: a response on behalf of the Council of the Association of Surgeons in Training. http://www.asit.org/assets/documents/ShoT%20Response%20Final%20Draft.pdf.
5. Couto TB, Kerrey BT, Taylor RG, FitzGerald M, Geis GL. Teamwork skills in actual, in situ, and in-center pediatric emergencies: performance levels across settings and perceptions of comparative educational impact. Simul Healthc. 2015;10(2):76–84.
6. Khan OA, McGlone ER, Mercer SJ, Somers SS, Toh SK. Outcomes following major emergency gastric surgery: the importance of specialist surgeons. Acta Chir Belg. 2015;115(2):131–5.
7. Sorensen JL, Thellesen L, Strandbygaard J, Svendsen KD, Christensen KB, Johansen M, et al. Development of knowledge tests for multi-disciplinary emergency training: a review and an example. Acta Anaesthesiol Scand. 2015;59(1):123–33.

Appendicitis

13

Gaetano Poillucci, Mauro Podda, Stavros Gourgiotis, and Salomone Di Saverio

13.1 Diagnostic Efficiency of Clinical Scoring Systems and Role of Imaging

Multiple diagnostic scoring systems have been developed with the aim to provide clinical probabilities that a patient has AA. These scores incorporate clinical features of the patient's history, physical examination, and laboratory parameters such as leukocyte count, neutrophils, and C-reactive protein level. Most popular and validated scoring systems in the daily clinical practice include the Alvarado score and the Appendicitis Inflammatory Response (AIR) score.

The Alvarado score performance is dependent on cut-off values. In terms of diagnostic accuracy, the cut-point of 5 is appropriate at ruling out admission for AA (sensitivity 99% overall, 96% men, 99% woman, 99% children). At the cut-point of 7, recommended for ruling in AA and progression to surgery, the score performs poorly (specificity overall 81%, men 57%, woman 73%, children 76%) [1]. Alvarado score of 9–10 shows 100% sensitivity to detect AA.

G. Poillucci (✉)
Department of Surgery "Paride Stefanini",
Policlinico Universitario Umberto I, Sapienza University, Rome, Italy

M. Podda
Emergency Surgery Unit, Department of Surgery,
Cagliari University Hospital "D.Casula", Cagliari, Italy

S. Gourgiotis
Department of Surgery, Addenbrooke's Hospital,
Cambridge University Hospitals, NHS Foundation Trust, Cambridge, UK
e-mail: stavros.gourgiotis@addenbrookes.nhs.uk

S. Di Saverio
Cambridge Colorectal Unit, Department of Surgery, Addenbrooke's Hospital,
Cambridge University Hospitals, NHS Foundation Trust, Cambridge, UK
e-mail: salomone.disaverio@addenbrookes.nhs.uk

© World Society of Emergency Surgery and Donegal Clinical and Research Academy 2020   95
M. Sugrue et al. (eds.), *Resources for Optimal Care of Emergency Surgery*,
Hot Topics in Acute Care Surgery and Trauma,
https://doi.org/10.1007/978-3-030-49363-9_13

The AIR score is based on eight variables: this score has shown a significant better discriminating capacity when compared with the Alvarado score, especially for advanced AA [2]. According to the AIR score, two cut-off points are identified to obtain three diagnostic test zones: a score < 4 (low probability) has a high sensitivity (96%) to rule out appendicitis; a score between 5 and 8 identifies the intermediate probability of AA, and suggests observation and eventual further imaging investigations; a score > 8 has a high specificity (99%) to rule in AA. The AIR score has demonstrated to be useful in guiding decision-making to reduce admissions, optimize utility of diagnostic imaging, and prevent negative surgical explorations (Table 13.1).

The decision to perform additional imaging for patients with suspected AA is based mainly on the complaints of the patient, combined with the findings at physical examination. Recent guidelines for diagnosis and treatment of AA state that the use of imaging techniques in the diagnostic workup should be linked to risk stratification such as Alvarado or AIR scores. Intermediate-risk classification identifies

Table 13.1 Clinical risk scores for suspected acute appendicitis: the Alvarado's and the AIR (Acute Inflammatory Response) scores

	Alvarado score	AIR score
Symptoms		
Nausea or vomiting	1	
Vomiting		1
Anorexia	1	
Migration of pain to the right lower quadrant	1	
Signs		
Pain in right lower quadrant	2	1
Rebound tenderness or muscular defense	1	
Light		1
Medium		2
Strong		3
Body temperature > 37.5 °C	1	
Body temperature > 38.5 °C		1
Laboratory tests		
Leucocytosis shift	1	
Polymorphonuclear leukocytes		
70–84%		1
≥85%		2
White blood cell count		
>10.0 × 10⁹/L	2	
10.0–14.9 × 10⁹/L		1
≥15.0 × 10⁹/L		2
C-reactive protein concentration		
10–49 g/L		1
≥50 g/L		2
Total score	*10*	*12*
Risk of appendicitis		
Alvarado score: 1–4	Alvarado score: 5–6	Alvarado score: 7–10
AIR score: 0–4	AIR score: 5–8	AIR score: 9–10
Low risk	Intermediate risk	High risk

Table 13.2 Imaging and diagnosis of acute appendicitis

Investigation	Diagnostic criteria	Evidence
Plain radiography	None	No role in diagnosis of acute appendicitis, although in some cases a fecalith may be shown
US	Aperistaltic and non-compressible structure with diameter > 6 mm	Sensitivity of 85%; specificity of 90%
CT scan	Abnormal appendix identified or calcified fecalith seen in association with periappendiceal inflammation or diameter > 6 mm	Sensitivity of 90–99%; specificity of 97%
MRI	Not confirmed	Restricted to cases in which radiation and diagnostic difficulties preclude use of other modalities (for example, pregnancy)

patients likely to benefit from systematic diagnostic imaging, whereas high-risk patients may not require preoperative imaging [3].

Ultrasonography (US) and Computed Tomography (CT) scans are the most effective methods for elucidating a diagnosis of AA. Depending on the operator, US has a sensitivity of approximately 85% and a specificity of 90%. Performing serial US may improve accuracy and reduce the use of CT scan. The use of CT imaging to diagnose AA has greatly affected the management of unclear cases. Depending on the radiologist skills, CT scan has a sensitivity of 90–99% and a specificity of 97%. In general, patients with a questionable history and physical who would have been observed closely in the past are now undergoing CT scan, and either being discharged or taken to the operating room. As clinicians become more comfortable with using CT scan as diagnostic tool, the rate of negative exploration is expected to decrease. Magnetic Resonance Imaging (MRI) is recommended in pregnant patients with suspected AA when US is inconclusive, and if the resource is available [3] (Table 13.2).

13.2   Timing of Appendectomy

Operative removal of the inflamed appendix is the accepted treatment for AA. Outcomes in relation to timing of surgery have been reported as controversial. Recently published studies have demonstrated no difference in outcome measures, including overall morbidity and serious morbidity or mortality between three groups of study (patients underwent appendectomy within 6 h, between 6 h and 12 h, and more than 12 h), thus demonstrating that delaying appendectomy for uncomplicated AA for up to 24 h after admission does not appear to be a risk factor for developing complicated AA, postoperative surgical-site infection or morbidity [4]. After the 24 h time period, the uncertainty of results in the literature is too large to draw any firm conclusions. For patients with clinical or radiological signs of complicated AA, delaying surgical treatment is not advocated.

13.3   Surgical Treatment

The appendix can be removed through an open incision or by laparoscopy. Laparoscopic Appendectomy (LA) nowadays represents, where technology and laparoscopic skills are available, the gold standard of treatment. Recent randomized controlled trials and meta-analyses confirmed that LA had significantly less surgical-site infections compared with Open Appendectomy (OA) [OR = 0.30], reduced time to oral intake [WMD = −0.98], and length of hospitalization [WMD = −3.49]. With regard to the incidence of intra-abdominal abscess, a recent cumulative meta-analysis of trials published up to and including 2001 demonstrated statistical significance in favor of OA (cumulative OR = 2.35). The effect size in favor of OA began to disappear after 2001, leading to an insignificant result with an overall cumulative OR of 1.32 when LA was compared with OA [5].

No significant difference in intra-abdominal abscess rates [OR = 1.11] has been detected even in another recent meta-analysis comparing LA and OA in adult patients with complicated AA [6] (Table 13.3).

If on the one hand LA is often associated with longer operative times (7.6–18.3 min) and higher operative costs, on the other hand, pain on day 1 is reduced after LA (by 8 mm on a 100 mm visual analog scale), thus allowing earlier return to normal daily activity and work.

On children the results do not seem to be much different when compared to adults. The main benefit of LA is that it can be helpful initially as a diagnostic tool and then the surgeon can proceed to appendectomy in positive cases, thus reducing the risk of a negative appendectomy.

This effect is stronger in fertile women as compared to unselected adults. LA offers clear advantages and should be preferred in obese patients (BMI > 30), patients older than 65 years (main advantages are shorter length of stay, mortality, and overall morbidity), and patients with comorbidities and with complicated AA (significant advantages include lower overall complications, readmission rate, small bowel obstruction rate, wound infections, faster recovery, and significantly lower overall costs). Laparoscopy should not be considered as first choice over OA in pregnant patients.

13.4   Role of Antibiotic Therapy

Recently, antibiotics have been proposed as first-line approach for uncomplicated AA.

Recently published RCTs reported an effectiveness of the conservative management with antibiotics of 65–85% at 1-year follow-up. Meta-analyses of RCTs comparing antibiotics and appendectomy have shown that, although antibiotic treatment alone can be successful, patients should be made aware of a failure rate at 1 year of

Table 13.3 Overview on meta-analyses comparing Laparoscopic (LA) and Open Appendectomy (OA) for AA published after 2000

Author	Year	Patients	IAA	Wound infections	Postoperative ileus	Overall complications	Operative time	LOS	Return to normal activity
Athanasiou C	2017	4439	Equivalent	LA superior	–	–	Equivalent	LA superior	LA superior
Dai L	2017	3642	Equivalent	LA superior	–	LA superior	OA superior	LA superior	LA superior
Yu MC	2017	142,905	Equivalent	LA superior	–	–	OA superior	LA superior	–
Ciarrocchi A	2014	57,900	Equivalent	LA superior	–	LA superior	LA superior	LA superior	–
Markar SR	2014	159,729	–	–	LA superior	–	–	–	–
Nataraja RM	2013	22,060	Equivalent	LA superior	LA superior	–	–	–	–
Markar SR	2012	34,474	OA superior	LA superior	–	LA superior	OA superior	LA superior	LA superior
Ohtani H	2012	5896	–	LA superior	–	–	LA superior	LA superior	–
Woodham BL	2012	2428	Equivalent	LA superior	–	LA superior	OA superior	LA superior	LA superior
Wei B	2011	4694	–	–	–	LA superior	OA superior	LA superior	LA superior
Li X	2010	5292	Equivalent	LA superior	Equivalent	Equivalent	OA superior	LA superior	LA superior
Liu Z	2010	3261	–	LA superior	Equivalent	Equivalent	OA superior	LA superior	LA superior
Markides G	2010	10,682	Equivalent	LA superior	–	–	OA superior	LA superior	–
Sauerland S	2010	5972	OA superior	LA superior	–	–	OA superior	LA superior	LA superior
Aziz O	2006	6477	Equivalent	LA superior	LA superior	–	Equivalent	LA superior	–
Sauerland S	2004	4953	OA superior	LA superior	–	–	OA superior	LA superior	LA superior

IAA postoperative intra-abdominal abscess, *LOS* postoperative length of hospital stay

around 25–30% with need for readmission or surgery. In the end, antibiotic therapy can be successful in selected patients with uncomplicated AA who wish to avoid surgery and accept the risk up to 38% recurrence. However, RCTs and meta-analyses have methodological limitations, including different criteria for diagnosis (some studies did not confirm diagnosis with imaging), inadequate outcome measures, and different length of follow-up between groups. For patients with equivocal clinical picture or imaging, or in those who have strong preferences for avoiding an operation, as well as in those patients with major comorbidities, an antibiotic-first challenge of up to 24 h is considered safe and feasible.

Employed antibiotic regimens should involve the use of antibiotics with aerobic and anaerobic coverage for ordinary bowel bacteria, taking into account local resistance patterns and the potential for heterogeneous causes. Current evidence supports initial intravenous antibiotics for 1–3 days, with subsequent switch to oral antibiotics. A reasonable recommendation is at least 1 day of intravenous treatment and hospital surveillance, with oral antibiotics subsequently given for 5–7 days [7] (Table 13.4).

13.5   Surgical Versus Non-surgical Treatment for Appendiceal Abscess

Preoperative intra-abdominal or pelvic abscess occurs in 3–8% of patients presenting with appendicitis and should be suspected in those presenting with a palpable mass. Although pre-hospital delay has traditionally been considered as a risk factor for perforation and abscess formation, evidence demonstrates that some patients might be at high risk of abscess formation despite prompt treatment. Conservative treatment (percutaneous drainage in addition to intravenous broad-spectrum antibiotics) is associated with significantly lower rates of overall complications (wound infections, abdominal/pelvic abscesses, ileus/bowel obstructions, and re-operations) when compared with immediate appendectomy [8]. However, newest evidence suggest that LA could be considered as a safe and effective alternative to non-operative management in presence of specific laparoscopic experience and advanced technical skills [9]. After successful conservative management, the indication to interval appendectomy is justified only in case of persistent or recurrent symptoms. On the contrary, appendectomy should be avoided in asymptomatic patients. Appendicular or colonic neoplasms should be investigated after conservatively treated abscesses, especially in patients older than 40 years: follow-up with colonoscopy, CT scan, or both is recommended.

Table 13.4 Summary of major outcomes reported in the randomized controlled trials comparing antibiotic treatment and appendectomy for uncomplicated AA published to date

Study and (year)		Eriksson S. (1995)	Styrud J. (2006)	Hansson J. (2009)	Turhan AN. (2009)	Vons C. (2011)	Salminen P. (2015)	Talan A. (2017)	Total (%)
No. of patients randomized	A	20	128	119	107	120	257	16	767
	S	20	124	250	183	119	273	14	983
Treatment efficacy based on 1 year follow-up (%)[a]	A	12 (60%)	113 (88.2%)	93 (78.2%)	88 (82.2%)	81 (68%)	186 (72.7%)	13 (81.3%)	586 (76.4%)
	S	17 (85%)	120 (96.8%)	223 (89.2%)	183 (100%)	117 (98.3%)	270 (98.9%)	12 (85.7%)	942 (95.8%)
Recurrence at 1 year follow-up (%)	A	7 (35%)	16 (15%)	15 (12.6%)	10 (9.3%)	44 (36.7%)	65 (25.3%)	2 (12.5%)	159 (20.7%)
	S	–	–	–	–	–	–	–	–
Complicated appendicitis identified at the time of the surgical operation, n (%)[b]	A	1 (14.3%)	12 (38.7%)	10 (8.4%)	–	9 (20.5%)	12 (17.1%)	–	44 (5.7%)
	S	1 (5%)	6 (5%)	42 (16.8%)	31 (16.9%)	21 (18%)	2 (0.7%)	4 (28.6%)	107 (10.9%)
Overall post-intervention complications (%)	A	0 (0%)	4 (3.1%)	3 (2.5%)	5 (4.7%)	12 (10%)	6 (2.3%)	1 (6.3%)	31 (4.1%)
	S	2 (10%)	17 (14%)	25 (10%)	8 (4.4%)	3 (2.5%)	49 (22.3%)	2 (14.3%)	106 (10.8%)

A antibiotics, *S* surgery (open/laparoscopic appendicectomy), *NR* not reported

[a]for surgical treatment (S), efficacy means positive diagnosis of acute appendicitis during operation and resolution of symptoms after surgical treatment

[b]in the antibiotic group, after failure of the primary treatment and subsequent surgery

References

1. Ohle R, O'Reilly F, O'Brien KK, Fahey T, Dimitrov BD. The Alvarado score for predicting acute appendicitis: a systematic review. BMC Med. 2011;9:139.
2. Andersson M, Andersson RE. The appendicitis inflammatory response score: a tool for the diagnosis of acute appendicitis that outperforms the Alvarado score. World J Surg. 2008;32(8):1843–9.
3. Di Saverio S, Birindelli A, Kelly MD, Catena F, Weber DG, Sartelli M, et al. WSES Jerusalem guidelines for diagnosis and treatment of acute appendicitis. World J Emerg Surg. 2016;11:34.
4. van Dijk ST, van Dijk AH, Dijkgraaf MG, Boermeester MA. Meta-analysis of in-hospital delay before surgery as a risk factor for complications in patients with acute appendicitis. Br J Surg. 2018;105(8):933–45.
5. Ukai T, Shikata S, Takeda H, Dawes L, Noguchi Y, Nakayama T, et al. Evidence of surgical outcomes fluctuates over time: results from a cumulative meta-analysis of laparoscopic versus open appendectomy for acute appendicitis. BMC Gastroenterol. 2016;16:37.
6. Athanasiou C, Lockwood S, Markides GA. Systematic review and meta-analysis of laparoscopic versus open appendicectomy in adults with complicated appendicitis: an update of the literature. World J Surg. 2017;41(12):3083–99.
7. Podda M, Cillara N, Di Saverio S, Lai A, Feroci F, Luridiana G, et al. Antibiotics-first strategy for uncomplicated acute appendicitis in adults is associated with increased rates of peritonitis at surgery. A systematic review with meta-analysis of randomized controlled trials comparing appendectomy and non-operative management with antibiotics. Surgeon. 2017;15(5):303–14.
8. Simillis C, Symeonides P, Shorthouse AJ, Tekkis PP. A meta-analysis comparing conservative treatment versus acute appendectomy for complicated appendicitis (abscess or phlegmon). Surgery. 2010;147(6):818–29.
9. Mentula P, Sammalkorpi H, Leppaniemi A. Laparoscopic surgery or conservative treatment for appendiceal abscess in adults? A randomized controlled trial. Ann Surg. 2015;262(2):237–42.

Acute Mesenteric Ischemia

14

Miklosh Bala and Jeffry Kashuk

14.1 Causes and Classification

An extensive mesenteric collateral network forms by the celiac artery (CA), superior mesenteric artery (SMA), and the inferior mesenteric artery (IMA). Of note, the SMA is affected in 85% of all cases of AMI. Accordingly, it plays the main role in the diagnosis of AMI [1]. The pathogenesis of the occlusion may be embolic or thrombotic, when in the presence of a pre-existing atheroma of the arterial wall. Often cited risk factors for AMI include cardiac arrhythmias, (mostly atrial fibrillation), older myocardial infarction, general arteriosclerosis, and arterial hypertension [2]. A separate type of a functional, non-occlusive mesenteric ischemia (NOMI) can occur in low-flow situations, e.g., at the end of cardiac surgery procedures or during dialysis [3].

14.1.1 Acute Mesenteric Arterial Ischemia

Acute mesenteric arterial ischemia results from arterial obstruction leading to conditions with varied clinical presentations [4].

1. *Embolic* occlusion of the SMA accounts for 40–50% of AMI [5]. Emboli usually originate in the heart but may come from proximal aortic atherosclerotic lesions as well. Typically, the proximal small bowel is spared due to the fact that the embolus typically lodges beyond the proximal portions of the SMA but the remainder of the small intestine and proximal colon are most commonly ischemic [6].

M. Bala (✉)
Hadassah—Hebrew University Medical Center, Jerusalem, Israel

J. Kashuk
Tel Aviv University Sackler School of Medicine, Tel Aviv, Israel

© World Society of Emergency Surgery and Donegal Clinical and Research Academy 2020   103
M. Sugrue et al. (eds.), *Resources for Optimal Care of Emergency Surgery*,
Hot Topics in Acute Care Surgery and Trauma,
https://doi.org/10.1007/978-3-030-49363-9_14

2. Acute *thrombosis* affects typically a principal mesenteric arterial vessel (20–35% of cases) [7]. Acute thrombosis of the SMA is most often secondary to an underlying proximal atherosclerotic lesion. In this setting, the majority of the small bowel and colon demonstrate ischemic changes, but the extent of necrosis will depend on the collateral circulation; which can be significant if the patient has suffered from long-standing atherosclerotic disease.

3. *Non-occlusive* mesenteric ischemia (NOMI) is typically associated with "low-flow states" and manifests with severe mesenteric vasoconstriction. The most common presentation of this entity is a patient in the intensive care unit who is critically ill, requiring vasopressor support, and develops evidence of increasing acidosis, abdominal pain or distension, and inability to tolerate enteral nutrition.

14.1.2 Acute Mesenteric Venous Thrombosis (AMVT)

Acute mesenteric venous thrombosis (AMVT) is a less common event (5–15%), and is most often related to the presence of an underlying hypercoagulable state [8]. Associated portal and splenic vein thrombosis may be part of the clinical picture.

Based on older autopsy data (1970–1980), SMA embolism was the most common cause of AMI with embolism-to-thrombosis ratio of 1.4:1 [9]. Of note, this distribution in 2000–2010 switched to 0.6:1 [10, 11]. Accordingly, atherosclerotic occlusive disease is currently the most common cause of AMI.

14.2 Pathophysiology and Clinical Aspects

Typically, SMA embolism is characterized by the acute onset of symptom, with the finding of severe abdominal pain without localization. "Pain out of proportion to clinical signs" is a common expression for this entity. In about 30% of the cases, the SMA embolus is located distal to the middle colic artery. In this scenario, rapid development of necrosis ensues; however, this leads to earlier detection and hence patients may survive, even without the need for revascularization.

The clinical presentation of AMI caused by mesenteric arterial thrombosis is typically more varied than in embolic AMI and reflects the extent of arterial obstruction and compensatory blood flow via collaterals. Patients with acute thrombotic occlusion of the SMA may present with fulminant bowel ischemia, or the symptoms may be unclear, including vague abdominal pain, diarrhea, and vomiting. Generally, in settings of atherosclerotic occlusive AMI the bowel may remain viable for longer periods of time. Of note, many of these patients may have suffered from prior chronic abdominal angina.

The potential clinical scenario in which NOMI is identified typically includes: severe heart failure, hypovolemia, sepsis, use of vasoconstrictive medications or intra-aortic balloon pump, hypotension caused by dialysis or major surgery (especially cardiac or aortic surgery), and abdominal compartment syndrome [12]. The clinical assessment of NOMI can be extremely challenging especially in patients that are intubated and mechanically ventilated in the intensive care unit.

In acute MVT, mild intestinal edema may gradually also contribute to arterial spasm and transmural bowel infarction within days to weeks. Abdominal pain in MVT most typically develops gradually within several weeks and may be mild, often times accompanied by diarrhea.

14.3 Diagnostic Examination

14.3.1 Laboratory Studies

The key to early diagnosis is a high index of clinical suspicion. Laboratory results are not conclusive but may help to support clinical suspicion. More than 90% of patients will have an abnormally elevated leukocyte count [13]. The second most commonly encountered abnormal finding is metabolic acidosis with elevated lactate level, which was noted in 88% [14].

Patients may present with early lactic acidosis due to dehydration alone. Accordingly, differentiation versus irreversible bowel injury based upon the lactate level alone is not reliable unless other clinical evidence exists [15]. It should be emphasized that the presence of lactic acidosis in combination with even mild abdominal pain in a patient who does not appear to be critically ill should prompt consideration for early CTA.

Unfortunately, there are currently no standardized blood tests that could be used widely in patients with acute abdominal pain to screen for AMI in such way as the troponin test is used for screening acute myocardial infarction in patients with acute chest pain. Of note, D-dimer has been reported to be important in diagnosis of intestinal ischemia, reflecting ongoing clot formation. No patient presenting with a normal D-dimer had intestinal ischemia and D-dimer >0.9 mg/L had a specificity, sensitivity, and accuracy of 82%, 60%, and 79%, respectively [16]. Similarly, hypercoagulable findings on thromboelastography may support the diagnosis, particularly if MVT has been suggested by imaging studies [17].

Potential biomarkers reported to assist in the diagnosis of AMI include intestinal fatty acid binding protein (I-FABP), serum alpha-glutathione S-transferase (alpha-GST), and cobalt-albumin binding assay (CABA) [17–19]. Further research is required to specify their potential use in the future.

In MVT laboratory tests are not helpful in making the diagnosis—they may neither confirm nor exclude the diagnosis—and should be used for screening purposes only. Other biochemical variables such as serum lactate and amylase may be not elevated [20].

14.3.2 Imaging/Computed Tomography Angiography (CTA)

Perhaps the most important management decision leading to early accurate diagnosis of AMI in all potential scenarios is CTA examination with accurate radiologic interpretation of images. CTA includes: (1) pre-contrast scans to detect vascular calcification, hyper-attenuating intravascular thrombus, and intramural hemorrhage; (2) arterial and venous phases which may demonstrate thrombus in the mesenteric arteries and veins, abnormal enhancement of the bowel wall and the presence of embolism or infarction of other organs; (3) sagittal reconstructions to assess the origin of the mesenteric arteries [21].

A sensitivity of 93%, specificity of 100%, and positive and negative predictive values of 100% and 94%, respectively, were achieved for the CT findings of visceral artery occlusion, intestinal pneumatosis, portomesenteric venous gas or bowel wall thickening in a recent studies [22, 23] (Fig. 14.1). In such a scenario, mandatory exploratory laparotomy should be performed to confirm the diagnosis and attempt surgical salvage.

In suspected NOMI, CTA will demonstrate bowel ischemia, free fluid but patent mesenteric vessels.

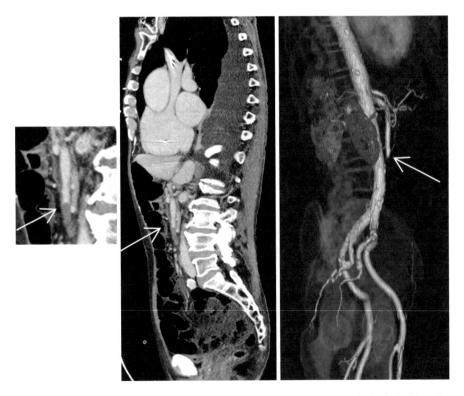

Fig. 14.1 84 year old male with atrial fibrillation presented with AMI. Embolus in SMA at the level of mid colic artery (arrow). 3D reconstruction clearly demonstrates distal occlusion of SMA

Fig. 14.2 56 year old patient with acute superior mesenteric vein thrombisis due to hypercoagulable state. SMV successfully treated with long-term anticoagulation

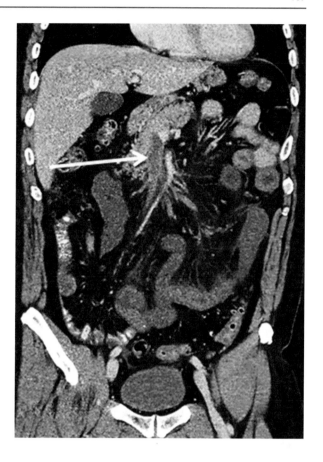

In MVT, the most common positive finding on venous phase of CTA is the demonstration of thrombus in the superior mesenteric vein (Fig. 14.2). Associated findings that may suggest MVT include bowel wall thickening, pneumatosis, and ascites. Portal or mesenteric venous gas strongly suggests the presence of bowel infarction. Duplex ultrasonography can be diagnostic only if obtained early and in chronic cases.

Contrast angiography has long been the gold standard for imaging the visceral vessels although it is now reserved for use in cases anticipating therapeutic intervention.

The risk of contrast-induced renal failure in patients with AMI is negligible especially if the patient has had normal kidney function before acute disease [24]. The acute kidney injury in AMI is usually caused by hypoperfusion, especially in NOMI. In some situations, the first images can be performed without contrast enhancement. Following this, in the absence of cholecystitis, appendicitis, diverticulitis, or pancreatitis, the examination should be continued with the use of contrast-enhanced protocol.

14.4   Treatment Strategy in AMI

14.4.1 General Considerations

AMI is a surgical emergency. Hemodynamically normal patients with abdominal pain or other risk factors suggestive of AMI should undergo prompt CTA, while the presence of peritonitis or shock mandate early abdominal exploration [13].

The modern treatment of AMI requires collaboration of general surgeons, vascular surgeons, and interventional radiologists. The treatment strategy is straightforward, targeting early restoration of blood flow to the intestine and bowel resection when appropriate, with consideration of the underlying etiology.

Fluid resuscitation of the patient with suspected AMI should parallel the diagnostic workup but not delay surgical intervention. The use of vasopressors in order to improve impaired hemodynamics should be avoided due to worsening of ischemia [3]. Broad-spectrum antibiotics (such as penicillin or a third-generation cephalosporin in combination with metronidazole) should be administered early because bowel ischemia, necrosis, and associated bacterial translocation are frequently noted [25].

Patients with AMI who have sepsis or septic shock and undergo life-saving surgery should have a damage control approach [26]. This includes immediate laparotomy with resection of ischemic bowel left in discontinuity, open thrombectomy (if indicated), and rapid transfer to the intensive care unit to continue resuscitation and physiologic restoration prior to embarking on definitive procedures, such as anastomosis and/or stoma [13]. This time frame may be 24–72 h, depending on the patient's individual response to therapy and subsequent stabilization. A temporary abdominal closure via a negative pressure wound therapy device should be considered, as these techniques have been shown to facilitate abdominal closure [27] via evacuation of abdominal ascites and early and continued wound traction.

14.4.2 Revascularization

14.4.2.1   Embolus to the Superior Mesenteric Artery

Surgical embolectomy remains the mainstay of therapy [28]. The procedure is usually performed via a midline incision approaching the SMA just below the pancreas at the mesenteric root. A transverse arteriotomy is then made after proximal and distal control and embolectomy catheters are used to clear the artery proximally and distally. After completing the thrombectomy, the artery should be flushed gently with heparinized saline. The arteriotomy is then closed primarily or with use of a venous patch. Full anticoagulation is required with continuous heparin (PTT goal of 70–80 s) followed by LMWH 1 mg/kg twice a day corrected to renal function.

Endovascular embolectomy may be achieved by percutaneous mechanical aspiration [29] or thrombolysis and permits percutaneous transluminal angioplasty (PTA), if necessary, with or without stenting [30–32]. The applicability of this approach is limited, since most patients present with symptoms that warrant an exploratory laparotomy for evaluation of intestinal viability.

14.4.2.2   SMA Thrombosis

Endovascular management is preferred for AMI thrombosis whenever possible and should be employed as expeditiously in order to minimize ongoing intestinal ischemia [33, 34]. If surgery is required for resection of ischemic/necrotic intestine, or when percutaneous treatment has failed, conventional arterial bypass surgery remains an important option [35]. There are a variety of bypass procedures, providing either antegrade or retrograde flow, with vein (preferably) or synthetic grafts. The most practical option for proximal mesenteric atherosclerotic occlusive disease is a retrograde bypass from the common iliac artery with a vein or synthetic graft.

14.4.2.3   NOMI

Management of NOMI is based on treatment of the underlying precipitating cause. Fluid resuscitation, optimization of cardiac output, and elimination of vasopressors remain important primary measures that improve outcome. Additional treatment may include systemic anticoagulation and the use of catheter-directed infusion of vasodilatory agents, most commonly papaverine hydrochloride [36]. The decision to intervene surgically is based on the presence of peritonitis, perforation, or overall worsening of the patient's condition. These patients are often in critical condition in the intensive care unit and mortality remains very high (50–85%) [37]. The key feature that should prompt the diagnosis of NOMI is the absence of occlusion of mesenteric vessels despite clinical suspicion of ischemia. These findings should assist in the difficult decision of taking a critically ill ICU patient to the operating room.

14.4.2.4   Venous Ischemia

MVT has a typical clinical finding on CT scan and when noted in a patient without findings of peritonitis, non-operative management may be considered. The first-line treatment for mesenteric venous thrombosis is anticoagulation. Systemic thrombolytic therapy is rarely indicated. When clinical signs demand operative intervention, only obvious necrotic bowel should be resected and damage control techniques use liberally, since anticoagulation therapy may rapidly improve the clinical picture over the ensuing 24–48 h. Early use of heparin has been associated with improved survival [38].

14.4.3   Revascularization: Open vs. Endovascular Techniques

The current ability to establish an early diagnosis of AMI via modern imaging techniques has prompted a current debate as to whether the primary treatment approach should be open or endovascular revascularization [39]. Clearly, the danger of endovascular techniques (EVT) is the risk of inadequate evaluation of bowel vitality and progression of necrosis. In contrast, however, laparotomy can be avoided by performing early and effective EVT [10, 40].

A PubMed search of studies published within the last 15 years treated with open, endovascular, or hybrid revascularization showed that EVT seems to perform at least equally, or better, as compared to open revascularization [28]. Of note, the outcome of any revascularization procedure in AMI is highly dependent on patient selection. In highly specialized centers, EVT proved technically successful in 88%. The 30-day mortality after successful or failed EVT was 32%, and the overall mortality of all 66 patients was 42%. Laparotomy was performed after EVT in 13 patients. Interestingly, only one-third of patients treated with EVT required bowel resection [40].

In the future, data from centers of excellence may help determine whether a hybrid operating theatre will provide an ideal solution to this difficult problem.

14.5 Postoperative Treatment and Follow-Up

Postoperative intensive care of AMI patients is directed towards the control of intestinal ischemia/reperfusion (I/R) and the prevention of a multiple organ failure (MOF) due to sepsis. Release of toxic products of local inflammatory processes can lead to MOF even in the absence of necrotic bowel. Capillary leakage resulting from I/R injury leads to volume sequestration into the third space. Therefore, particular attention is required regarding the optimization of metabolic status. Systemic hypotension often requires catecholamine administration.

In such a scenario, depending on cardiac output and peripheral vascular resistance, a combination of noradrenaline and dobutamine should be considered to minimize the possible negative impact on the intestinal microcirculation [41]. Dialysis, which is often required because of associated acute kidney injury, may contribute to hemodynamic stabilization and facilitate optimization of fluid balance.

Because of potential bacterial translocation from the injured gut, broad-spectrum antibacterial treatment according to current guidelines should always be initiated [42]. Systemic heparin is administered postoperatively (with goal activated Partial Thromboplastin Time (aPTT) between 40 and 60) in all patients. If preferred, low-molecular weight heparin (LMWH) in therapeutic doses is a good alternative.

Enteral feeding is preferred, but some patients may need parenteral nutrition for a prolonged time based upon gut status.

Virtually all patients with AMI will require lifelong antiplatelet therapy to prevent concurrent or subsequent atherosclerosis [43]. In patients following endovascular stent placement, clopidogrel is administered for 6 months and acetylsalicylic acid as lifelong maintenance treatment.

Continued patient surveillance for the development of stent or graft restenosis is important, as AMI after mesenteric revascularization accounts for 6–8% of late deaths [44]. It is important to emphasize that the optimal technology for stent placement in AMI has not yet been achieved. Accordingly, clinical evaluation with duplex imaging should be performed due to current evidence for high restenosis rate for stents in the first 2 years [45]. If further suspicion exists, CTA should then be performed.

14.6 Summary

AMI is a multifactorial syndrome, caused most commonly by arterial insufficiency (thrombosis or embolism) or less commonly by venous obstruction. NOMI occurs with splanchnic vasoconstriction, which can be caused by hypovolemia, hypotension, decreased cardiac output and exogenous vasopressors.

While a definitive diagnosis of acute mesenteric ischemia may often be elusive, particularly in a critically ill patient, a high index of suspicion based upon laboratory, clinical findings, or even vague abdominal pain should prompt early diagnostic imaging which has a high degree of accuracy and can help guide subsequent decision-making.

Specialized centers have advocated endovascular procedures for prompt mesenteric revascularization, although open evaluation of the bowel should not be delayed if there is any evidence of prior or ongoing ischemia. In patients with arterial embolism, options include endovascular aspiration, mechanical embolectomy, and local thrombolysis.

Prompt surgical management of AMI is the current standard approach. The damage control techniques and continued critical care resuscitation has no doubt contributed to the salvage of increasing critically ill patients.

Anticoagulation is the treatment of choice for venous thrombosis while lifelong antiplatelet therapy is indicated in cases of AMI with underlying arterial atherosclerotic disease.

A multidisciplinary approach with close cooperation between acute care surgeons, radiologists, and vascular surgeons may assist early diagnosis and subsequent improved survival for patients with AMI.

References

1. Rosenblum JD, Boyle CM, Schwartz LB. The mesenteric circulation. Anatomy and physiology. Surg Clin North Am. 1997;77:289–306.
2. Bala M, Kashuk J. Acute mesenteric ischemia. Acute care surgery handbook. Vol 2. New York: Springer; 2016.
3. Sise MJ. Mesenteric ischemia: the whole spectrum. Scand J Surg. 2010;99:106–10.
4. Corcos O, Nuzzo A. Gastro-intestinal vascular emergencies. Best Pract Res Clin Gastroenterol. 2013;27:709–25.
5. Vokurka J, Olejnik J, Jedlicka V, Vesely M, Ciernik J, Paseka T. Acute mesenteric ischemia. Hepato-Gastroenterology. 2008;55:1349–52.
6. Ottinger LW. The surgical management of acute occlusion of the superior mesenteric artery. Ann Surg. 1978;188:721–31.
7. Oldenburg WA, Lau LL, Rodenberg TJ, Edmonds HJ, Burger CD. Acute mesenteric ischemia: a clinical review. Arch Intern Med. 2004;164:1054–62.

8. Kumar S, Sarr MG, Kamath PS. Mesenteric venous thrombosis. N Engl J Med. 2001;345:1683–8.
9. Acosta S. Epidemiology of mesenteric vascular disease: clinical implications. Semin Vasc Surg. 2010;23:4–8.
10. Ryer EJ, Kalra M, Oderich GS, Duncan AA, Gloviczki P, Cha S, et al. Revascularization for acute mesenteric ischemia. J Vasc Surg. 2012;55:1682–9.
11. Lehtimaki TT, Karkkainen JM, Saari P, Manninen H, Paajanen H, Vanninen R. Detecting acute mesenteric ischemia in CT of the acute abdomen is dependent on clinical suspicion: review of 95 consecutive patients. Eur J Radiol. 2015;84:2444–53.
12. Kolkman JJ, Mensink PB. Non-occlusive mesenteric ischaemia: a common disorder in gastro-enterology and intensive care. Best Pract Res Clin Gastroenterol. 2003;17:457–73.
13. Bala M, Kashuk J, Moore EE, Kluger Y, Biffl W, Gomes CA, Ben-Ishay O, Rubinstein C, Balogh ZJ, Civil I, Coccolini F, Leppaniemi A, Peitzman A, Ansaloni L, Sugrue M, Sartelli M, Di Saverio S, Fraga GP, Catena F. Acute mesenteric ischemia: guidelines of the World Society of Emergency Surgery. World J Emerg Surg. 2017;12:38.
14. Kougias P, Lau D, El Sayed HF, Zhou W, Huynh TT, Lin PH. Determinants of mortality and treatment outcome following surgical interventions for acute mesenteric ischemia. J Vasc Surg. 2007;46:467–74.
15. Nuzzo A, Maggiori L, Ronot M, Becq A, Plessier A, Gault N, Joly F, Castier Y, Vilgrain V, Paugam C, Panis Y, Bouhnik Y, Cazals-Hatem D, Corcos O. Predictive factors of intestinal necrosis in acute mesenteric ischemia: prospective study from an intestinal stroke center. Am J Gastroenterol. 2017;112:597–605.
16. Block T, Nilsson TK, Björck M, Acosta S. Diagnostic accuracy of plasma biomarkers for intestinal ischaemia. Scand J Clin Lab Invest. 2008;68:242–8.
17. Kashuk JL, Moore EE, Sabel A, Barnett C, Haenel J, Le T, Pezold M, Lawrence J, Biffl WL, Cothren CC, Johnson JL. Rapid thrombelastography (r-TEG) identifies hypercoagulability and predicts thromboembolic events in surgical patients. Surgery. 2009;146:764–72.
18. Matsumoto S, Sekine K, Funaoka H, Yamazaki M, Shimizu M, Hayashida K, Kitano M. Diagnostic performance of plasma biomarkers in patients with acute intestinal ischaemia. Br J Surg. 2014;101:232–8.
19. Treskes N, Persoon AM, van Zanten ARH. Diagnostic accuracy of novel serological biomark-ers to detect acute mesenteric ischemia: a systematic review and meta-analysis. Intern Emerg Med. 2017;12:821–36.
20. Russell CE, Wadhera RK, Piazza G. Mesenteric venous thrombosis. Circulation. 2015;131:1599–603.
21. Furukawa A, Kanasaki S, Kono N, Wakamiya M, Tanaka T, Takahashi M, Murata K. CT diag-nosis of acute mesenteric ischemia from various causes. Am J Roentgenol. 2009;192:408–16.
22. Hagspiel KD, Flors L, Hanley M, Norton PT. Computed tomography angiography and mag-netic resonance angiography imaging of the mesenteric vasculature. Tech Vasc Interv Radiol. 2015;18:2–13.
23. Oliva IB, Davarpanah AH, Rybicki FJ, et al. ACR Appropriateness criteria imaging of mesen-teric ischemia. Abdom Imaging. 2013;38:714–9.
24. Acosta S, Bjornsson S, Ekberg O, Resch T. CT angiography followed by endovascular inter-vention for acute superior mesenteric artery occlusion does not increase risk of contrast-induced renal failure. Eur J Vasc Endovasc Surg. 2010;39:726–30.
25. Corcos O, Castier Y, Sibert A, et al. Effects of a multimodal management strategy for acute mesenteric ischemia on survival and intestinal failure. Clin Gastroenterol Hepatol. 2013;11:158–65.
26. Weber DG, Bendinelli C, Balogh ZJ. Damage control surgery for abdominal emergencies. Br J Surg. 2014;101:e109–18.
27. Roberts DJ, Zygun DA, Grendar J, Ball CG, Robertson HL, Ouellet J-F, Cheatham ML, Kirkpatrick AW. Negative-pressure wound therapy for critically ill adults with open abdominal wounds: a systematic review. J Trauma Acute Care Surg. 2012;73:629–39.

28. Kärkkäinen JM, Acosta S. Acute mesenteric ischemia (Part II)—vascular and endovascular surgical approaches. Best Pract Res Clin Gastroenterol. 2017;31:27–38.
29. Kim BG, Ohm JY, Bae MN, Kim HN, Kim YJ, Chung MH, Park CS, Ihm SH, Kim HY. Successful percutaneous aspiration thrombectomy for acute mesenteric ischemia in a patient with atrial fibrillation despite optimal anticoagulation therapy. Can J Cardiol. 2013;29:1329.e5–7.
30. Jia Z, Jiang G, Tian F, Zhao J, Li S, Wang K, Wang Y, Jiang L, Wang W. Early endovascular treatment of superior mesenteric occlusion secondary to thromboemboli. Eur J Vasc Endovasc Surg. 2014;47:196–203.
31. Yanar F, Agcaoglu O, Sarici IS, Sivrikoz E, Ucar A, Yanar H, et al. Local thrombolytic therapy in acute mesenteric ischemia. World J Emerg Surg. 2013;8:8.
32. Raupach J, Lojik M, Chovanec V, Renc O, Strýček M, Dvořák P, et al. Endovascular management of acute embolic occlusion of the superior mesenteric artery: a 12-year single-centre experience. Cardiovasc Interv Radiol. 2016;39:195–203.
33. Blauw JTM, Meerwaldt R, Brusse-Keizer M, Kolkman JJ, Gerrits D, Geelkerken RH. Retrograde open mesenteric stenting for acute mesenteric ischemia. J Vasc Surg. 2014;60:726–34.
34. Beaulieu RJ, Arnaoutakis KD, Abularrage CJ, Efron DT, Schneider E, Black JH III. Comparison of open and endovascular treatment of acute mesenteric ischemia. J Vasc Surg. 2014;59:159–64.
35. Tilsed JV, Casamassima A, Kurihara H, Mariani D, Martinez I, Pereira J, Ponchietti L, Shamiyeh A, Al-Ayoubi F, Barco LA, Ceolin M, D'Almeida AJ, Hilario S, Olavarria AL, Ozmen MM, Pinheiro LF, Poeze M, Triantos G, Fuentes FT, Sierra SU, Soreide K, Yanar H. ESTES guidelines: acute mesenteric ischaemia. Eur J Trauma Emerg Surg. 2016;42:253–70.
36. Boley SJ, Sprayregan S, Siegelman SS, Veith FJ. Initial results from an aggressive roentgenological and surgical approach to acute mesenteric ischemia. Surgery. 1977;82:848–55.
37. Schoots IG, Koffeman GI, Legemate DA, Levi M, van Gulik TM. Systematic review of survival after acute mesenteric ischaemia according to disease aetiology. Br J Surg. 2004;91:17–27.
38. Abdu RA, Zakhour BJ, Dallis DJ. Mesenteric venous thrombosisd1911 to 1984. Surgery. 1987;101:383–8.
39. Bjorck M, Orr N, Endean ED. Debate: whether an endovascular-first strategy is the optimal approach for treating acute mesenteric ischemia. J Vasc Surg. 2015;62:767–72.
40. Kärkkäinen JM, Lehtimaki TT, Saari P, Hartikainen J, Rantanen T, Paajanen H, et al. Endovascular therapy as a primary revascularization modality in acute mesenteric ischemia. Cardiovasc Interv Radiol. 2015;38:1119–29.
41. Luther B, Mamopoulos A, Lehmann C, Klar E. The ongoing challenge of acute mesenteric ischemia. Visc Med. 2018;34:217–23.
42. Rhodes A, Evans LE, Alhazzani W, Levy MM, Antonelli M, Ferrer R, Kumar A, Sevransky JE. Surviving sepsis campaign: international guidelines for management of sepsis and septic shock: 2016. Intensive Care Med. 2017;43:304–77.
43. Clair DG, Beach JM. Mesenteric ischemia. N Engl J Med. 2016;374:959–68.
44. Tallarita T, Oderich GS, Gloviczki P, Duncan AA, Kalra M, Cha S, et al. Patient survival after open and endovascular mesenteric revascularization for chronic mesenteric ischemia. J Vasc Surg. 2013;57:747–55.
45. Bjornsson S, Resch T, Acosta S. Symptomatic mesenteric atherosclerotic disease-lessons learned from the diagnostic workup. J Gastrointest Surg. 2013;17:97–80.

Intra-abdominal Hypertension and Abdominal Compartment Syndrome: Updates

15

Bruno M. Pereira and Pablo R. Ottolino-Lavarte

15.1 Introduction

The abdominal compartment syndrome (ACS) is a serious complication derived from the exaggerated increase of the intra-abdominal pressure (IAP), causing significant morbidity and mortality. The pathophysiological alterations derived from the increase in IAP in several organs and systems have been studied since the last century, initially to emphasize the cardiovascular consequence associated with the elevation of the IAP. However, recognition of the abdominal cavity as a compartment and the concept that intra-abdominal hypertension (IAH) results in ACS have recently received more attention. The clinical severity and the frequency of the IAH/ACS justify attention to this topic [1].

ACS is defined as a symptomatic organic dysfunction that results from increased intra-abdominal pressure. The term ACS was coined by Fietsam in 1989 after describing the picture of a patient in postoperative recovery of abdominal aortic aneurysm that evolved with tense abdomen, oliguria, hypoxemia, hypercarbia, and high peak inspiratory pressure. Subsequently, the IAP measurement became available and clinical studies ended up demonstrating the low sensitivity of the physical examination, making the measurement method through the intra-vesical pressure (bladder) standard in most trauma centers and intensive care units worldwide [2, 3].

The incidence of IAH has not been well studied and there is a lack of prospective, double-blind, randomized and evidence-based analyses. If the ACS is a serious

B. M. Pereira (✉)
Vassouras University, Vassouras, RJ, Brazil

Grupo Surgical - Acute Care Surgery, Campinas, Brazil

P. R. Ottolino-Lavarte
Emergency and Trauma Unit, Hospital Sótero del Rio, Santiago del Chile, Santiago, Chile

© World Society of Emergency Surgery and Donegal Clinical and Research Academy 2020   115
M. Sugrue et al. (eds.), *Resources for Optimal Care of Emergency Surgery*,
Hot Topics in Acute Care Surgery and Trauma,
https://doi.org/10.1007/978-3-030-49363-9_15

consequence of the elevation of the IAP, it is necessary to better understand some basic concepts. By definition, IAP is the pressure contained inside the abdominal compartment. Although physiologically the IAP can reach transient marks of up to 80 mmHg (cough, Valsalva maneuver, weight lifting, etc.), these values cannot be tolerated for long periods of time. According to the World Society of the Abdominal Compartment (WSACS) [4], founded in 2004 and responsible for the most recent studies on the subject, critical adult patients already have an increased IAP (5–7 mmHg). IAH in turn is defined as an IAP above 12 mmHg. The harmful effects of IAH occur long before the manifestation of ACS and patients presenting with IAH are associated with an increase in abdominal complications 11 times greater than those without IAH/ACS [1, 2, 4].

Thus, the rapid progression of IAH leads to ACS which is formally defined as IAP > 20 mmHg. ACS should, therefore, be seen as the final result of a continuous and progressive increase of the IAP and that if not corrected will result in the dysfunction or failure of multiple organs [2, 4]. Here are the following common causes of dysfunction/multiple organ failure:

- Metabolic acidosis (due to volemic resuscitation).
- Oliguria.
- Pressure of the raised airways.
- Hypercarbons refractory to increased respiratory rate.
- Hypoxemia refractory to oxygen and PEEP.
- Intracranial hypertension.

The global consensus of definitions of IAP/IAH/ACS developed by WSACS can be seen briefly in the following table (Table 15.1).

Table 15.1 Definitions recommended by WSACS

Definition 1: Intra-abdominal pressure is by definition the pressure contained within the abdominal compartment.
Definition 2: Abdominal perfusion pressure = mean arterial pressure − intra-abdominal pressure (APP = IAP − MAP).
Definition 3: Filtration Gradient (FG) = Glomerular filtration pressure (GFP) − proximal tubular pressure (PTP) = MAP − (2 × PIA).
Definition 4: Measurement of IAP will be measured in mmHg, supine position and expiration after verification that there is no contraction of the abdominal wall and that the transducer is "zero" at the level of the median axillary line.
Definition 5: The measurement of the IAP should be made through intra-vesical pressure with a maximum instillation of 25 ml of the sterile saline solution.
Definition 6: The IAP can be considered normal at approximately 5–7 mmHg in critical patients.
Definition 7: IAH is defined by sustained or repeated IAP ≥ 12 mmHg.
Definition 8: IAH is classified in Grade I: PIA 12–15 mmHg, Grade II: PIA 16–20 mmHg, Grade III: PIA 21–25 mmHg, Grade IV: PIA > 25 mmHg.
Definition 9: ACS is defined by sustained or repeated IAP ≥20 mmHg (with or without perfusion pressure < 60 mmHg) that is associated with organ dysfunction or failure.

Table 15.1 (continued)

Definition 10: Primary ACS is the condition associated with the lesion or disease located within the abdominopelvic cavity.

Definition 11: Secondary ACS refers to the condition in which the etiology does not originate from the abdominopelvic region.

Definition 12: Tertiary or recurrent ACS is the condition in which there is recurrence of ACS after surgical intervention or prior clinical treatment of primary or secondary ACS.

15.2   Etiology and Physiopathology

Any abnormality that induces the elevation of pressure inside the abdominal cavity can lead to IAH. In most cases, the potential causes of IAH and ACS include: acute pancreatitis, abdominal aortic aneurysm, abdominal and retroperitoneal tumors, metabolic ileus, mechanical obstruction of the bowel, trauma, massive transfusion, sepsis [3–5].

Trauma, mainly those scenarios with intra-abdominal hemorrhage that results from spleen, liver, and mesentery injuries are the most common causes of IAH/ACS. However, in situations where damage control surgery is necessary, the use of lap pads in the abdominal cavity also increases intra-abdominal pressure as well as distention and edema of the bowel loops. Hypovolemic shock, exacerbated volemic replacement, and massive transfusion are important and well-known causes of IAH/ACS, related to trauma. Sepsis has also become another high incident cause of IAH.

In the states of hypovolemic shock, vasoconstriction mediated by the sympathetic nervous system decreases blood flow to the skin, muscles, kidneys, and gastrointestinal tract in favor of perfusion of the heart and brain. This physiological defense mechanism ends up producing cellular hypoxia. The hypoxia generated in the intestinal tissue resulting from the marked reduction of splanchnic circulation is associated with three crucial factors for the development of the vicious cycle that characterizes the pathogenesis of IAH and its progression towards ACS [6]:

1. Cytokine release.
2. Formation of oxygen free radicals.
3. Decreased cell production of adenosine triphosphate (ATP).

In response to tissue hypoxic injury, pro-inflammatory cytokines are released. These molecules promote vasodilation and increase capillary permeability, leading to the formation of edema. After cellular reperfusion, oxygen free radicals are generated and have a toxic effect on cell membranes, aggravated by the presence of cytokines, which stimulate the release of more free radicals. In addition, the insufficient supply of oxygen to tissues limits the production of ATP, damaging all activities dependent on cellular energy, particularly sodium and potassium pumps. The

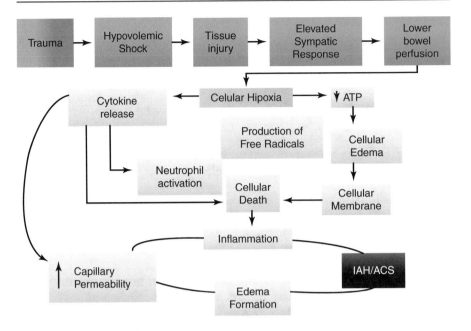

Fig. 15.1 Vicious cycle of IAH

efficient functioning of the Na+/K+ pump is essential for the intracellular regulation of electrolytes. When the pump fails, there is a flow of sodium and water in the cells. With cellular edema, the membranes lose their integrity, spilling intracellular content for the extracellular environment, promoting tissue irritation and inflammation. Inflammation in turn rapidly leads to the formation of edema, as a result of capillary enlargement and fragility promoting for example edema of intestinal braces and increase of IAP. With increased IAP, the abdominal perfusion pressure (APP) decreases and the cycle—cellular hypoxia, inflammation, edema, and cell death perpetuate (Fig. 15.1) [3–6].

15.3   Clinical Manifestations

The alteration of the IAP has important systemic effects. From now on we will see in detail the effects of the IAH in different organs and systems; however two essential points musr be emphasized: 1) the measurement of intra-vesical IAP (current pattern) is essential for the diagnosis of this complication and 2) physical examination alone is not accuarate for the diagnosis of IAH/ACS. Recent research has shown that the sensitivity of the physical examination in the presence of ACS varies between 40 and 61% and that the positive predictive value varies between 45 and 76%. In this way we can conclude that the possibility of diagnosing the ACS through the physical examination only is the same (or less) than playing a coin up betting on one of the faces, that is, 50% (or less) [1–4, 6].

15.4   Effects of HIA on Different Organs and Systems [7]

15.4.1 Cerebral Perfusion

The altered cerebral perfusion pressure (CPP) was described in morbidly obese patients with chronic IAH. The increase in IAP forces the diaphragm upwards decreasing the volume of the thoracic cavity and increasing the intrathoracic pressure (ITP). Increased ITP leads to increased jugular venous pressure and hinders the venous return of the brain, in turn raising intracranial pressure (ICP) and consequently, decreasing cerebral blood flow. These alterations are not unusual in the immediate postoperative period and IAH/ACS can make the CPP even worse in cases of trauma patients with abdominal injuries combined with brain injuries.

15.4.2 Cardiac Function

IAH hinders venous return, even causing edema of the lower limbs. High ITP virtually elevates central venous pressure (CVP) and pulmonary artery pressure (PAP). At the same time, the post-loading pressure of the left ventricle rises due to increased vascular resistance. Elevated ITP also increases the right ventricular afterload, which when extremely high, causes right ventricular failure and dilatation with consequent deviation of the cardiac septum to the left, making it difficult to fill the left ventricle. Clinically, the patient presents with low cardiac output, high filling pressures, and high peripheral vascular resistance.

15.4.3 Respiratory Function

The elevation of the IAP decreases chest compliance and the higher pressures are necessary for adequate mechanical ventilation. In addition, the residual functional capacity is also reduced and the ventilation perfusion ratio increases, causing difficult exchange and difficult oxygenation. Clinically, it is a patient "difficult to ventilate and oxygenate."

15.4.4 Renal Function

Oliguria or anuria in spite of the aggressive volemic replacement is a typical sign of ACS, described by some authors as the first clinical sign that appears in the presence of IAH. The mechanisms responsible for the decrease in renal function include direct compression of the renal parenchyma, decreased renal perfusion due to decreased cardiac output and water retention and sodium caused by the activation of the renin-angiotensin system. It is very important to interpret the volume of urine output in the context and magnitude of the volumetric resuscitation instead of relying on relatively normal absolute numbers only.

15.4.5 Intestinal Function

IAH impairs splanchnic perfusion due to decreased cardiac output and increased peripheral and splanchnic vascular resistance. When severe, tissue ischemia can occur.

15.4.6 Peripheral Perfusion

The elevation of the IAP increases femoral venous pressure and peripheral vascular resistance, and reduces femoral arterial flow by up to 65%.

Compartment syndrome of extremities due to trauma, volemic resuscitation or reperfusion syndrome are common risk factor for the development of ACS [7, 8].

Table 15.2 shows the main clinical manifestations derived from the IAH/ACS.

15.5 Classification of IAH/ACS

Table 15.3 below shows the classification of IAH advocated by WSACS [4].

ACS can be classified as primary ACS, secondary ACS, and tertiary or recurrent ACS.

Primary ACS is the condition associated with trauma or abdominopelvic disease that often requires early surgical intervention or radiological intervention

Table 15.2 Clinical manifestations of the IAH/ACS

Central nervous system
- Elevation of the ICP
- Decrease in CPP

Cardiovascular system
- Hypovolemia
- Decrease in cardiac output
- Decreased venous return
- Increase in PAP and CVP
- Increase in peripheral vascular resistance

Respiratory system
- Elevation of the ITP
- Increase in ventilatory pressures
- Decrease in thoracic compliance
- Change of ventilation/perfusion ratio

Digestive system
- Decreased splanchnic blood flow
- Mucosal ischemia and increased bacterial translocation

Urinary system
- Decreased urinary flow
- Decreased renal perfusion
- Decrease in glomerular filtration rate

Abdominal wall
- Decrease in abdominal compliance

Table 15.3 Classification of the HIA

Grade I	IAH 12–15 mmHg IAH
Grade II	IAH 16–20 mmHg IAH
Grade III	IAH 21–25 mmHg IAH
Grade IV	IAH > 25 mmHg

(interventional radiology) (Table 15.1, definition) [10]. Examples are: abdominal and pelvic tumors, abdominal trauma, ascites.

Secondary ACS refers to conditions that are not native to the abdominopelvic topography, for example, sepsis, massive volemic resuscitation, and large burns (grade III abdominal burns).

Tertiary or recurrent ACS refers to the requirement in which ACS resurfaces after clinical/surgical treatment of primary or secondary ACS [3–5, 9, 10].

15.6   Diagnosis and Management of the IAH/ACS

The diagnosis of ACS should be made by measuring intra-vesical pressure. In accordance with the configurations recommended by WSACS, the pressure scale used must be in mmHg. As in some of the hospital services in the Americas, the pressure scale used is in cmH_2O and the conversion of the pressure scales must therefore be carried out. Conversion websites are available on the Internet or in general, dividing the value in cmH_2O by 1.36 results in the approximate value in mmHg. The value of the IAP that induces the multiple failure of organs is variant for each patient; in this way, the calculation of the APP must be performed in all patients who had the IAP measured and converted into mmHg (APP = IAP − MAP). The APP is the most reliable variant to determine the degree of perfusion of the abdominal organs. Thus APP > IAP > arterial pH > Base Deficit > lactate in the prediction of multiple organ failure and prognosis. Failure to maintain the APP >60 mmHg in the first 3 days after diagnosis represents a decrease in the prognosis of these patients [11, 12]. Special attention must be given when calculating APP in patients on vasoactive drug high dose use. Clinical experience shows that some bias on APP value might be present when facing this scenario; however, no evidence-based data are available yet.

The risk factors associated with the presence of IAH and ACS are important predictors for the presence of this co-morbidity and should be evaluated in the admission of the patient at the emergency room/ICU or in the presence of organic dysfunction. Common risk factors are among others: [12–14].

- Trauma/lethal triad (hypotension, coagulopathy, and acidosis).
- Multiple blood transfusions/High volume of crystalloid infusion (>3.5 L/24 h) or Sepsis.
- Alterations of the intra-abdominal volume.
- Pulmonary, renal, and/or hepatic dysfunction or metabolic ileum.
- Abdominal Surgery/Synthesis of the abdominal aponeurosis.

In the presence of two or more risk factors, the IAP should be measured. In the presence of IAH, the serial measurement of the IAP must be performed in all critical phases of the patient. It is very important that each service has adapted its reality to a measurement protocol of the IAP based on the guidelines of the WSACS [2, 4]. To date, IAP should be looked as a new vital sign that helps on management of critical ill patients.

Intra-abdominal pressure is an important physiological parameter that is often still neglected by the medical community. It should be measured regularly in critically ill patients, from 4 to 6 h, according to guidelines [2–4]. A missed IAH diagnosis can lead to a longer stay in the ICU, prolonged ventilation and a higher incidence of ventilator associated pneumonia (VAP), among other indirect consequences that affect the patient's recovery. Therefore, it is essential that doctors and nurses in the ICU are aware of the importance of IAH and ACS in both adults and children. The presence of one or more risk factors for IAH should promote adequate IAP monitoring and help facilitate early diagnosis. As mentioned, this monitoring should be included as a vital sign in the daily clinical evaluation of all critically ill patients.

Recently, the WSACS developed a medical management algorithm with a gradual approach based on the evolution of intra-abdominal pressure in order to maintain the IAP ≤15 mmHg (level of evidence grade 1C) [15, 16]. This algorithm is based on five basic principles:

1. Evacuation of intraluminal contents (e.g., feces, residual gastric volume).
2. Evacuation of intra-abdominal contents (e.g., abscess, blood draw, ascites).
3. Improvement of compliance of the abdominal wall.
4. Optimization of fluid administration (neutral fluid balance).
5. Optimization of systemic and regional perfusion.

With the increased use of ultrasound as a bedside modality in both emergency patients and critical patients, the WSACS also created an addendum in a new publication inserting the use of bedside ultrasonography (POCUS) in the preparatory protocol of the IAH/ACS [15]. This may be particularly relevant for the first and second basic stages of the algorithm.

When the ultrasonography apparatus is used, the transducer should be placed as shown in Fig. 15.2 to look for the following elements shown in the flow diagram of Fig. 15.3.

The measurement technique of the IAP is simple and economically accessible for hospitals. When it is not measured in a water column intermittently from 6 to 6 h, other technologies already allow the continuous measurement of the IAP through the connection of the pressure transducer cable in the cardiac monitor (Abthera, ConvaTec, USA).

The basic principles essential to the management of the IAH/ACS are:

1. Continued IAP measurement.
2. Optimization of systemic perfusion and organic function.
3. Institution of specific clinical interventions for control and reduction of the IAP.
4. Immediate surgical decompression for IAP refractory to the previous measures.

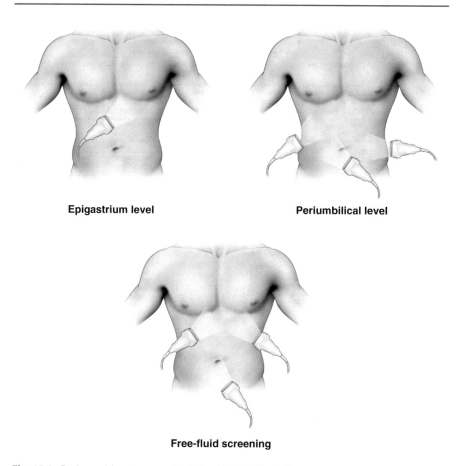

Epigastrium level   **Periumbilical level**

Free-fluid screening

Fig. 15.2 Probe position to access the different POCUS windows

Based on the basic principles described above, in the presence of IAH, the clinical measures should be used to objectify the impediment of the growing evolution of the IAP and the improvement of the picture. The WSACS offers on its website the strategies and measures applicable in the clinical management of the IAH, measures increasingly recognized as important factors in the prevention and treatment of this aforementioned complication [4].

Actions such as reducing the tone of the thoracoabdominal musculature with sedation, analgesia, and neuromuscular block potentially reduce the IAP to lower levels and therefore are important clinical measures to be taken in the care of the critical patient with the diagnosis of IAH. In the literature, prospective studies are not available evaluating the risks and benefits of sedation and analgesia in IAH/ACS. These measures described above are, in fact, possible adjuncts in the control of the IAH based on current knowledge of the pathophysiology of this co-morbidity [17].

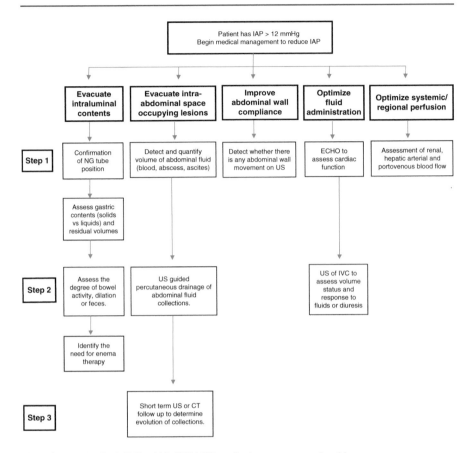

Fig. 15.3 Role of POCUS within WSACS medical management algorithm

The use of nasogastric tube, enemas, and endoscopic decompression are other simple and minimally invasive methods used to reduce IAP and treat IAH grades I, II, and eventually III in a sub-acute scenario and that does not imply risk of immediate death. Gastrointestinal motility stimulating agents have not yet demonstrated reliable evidence on their effects on the evacuation of the intraluminal content of the intestine and consequent reduction of the total volume of the viscera, but they are routinely used by various services.

Once the primary ACS is diagnosed, the gold-standard treatment established is surgical decompression through a medium-sized pubertal laparotomy [18]. Once the damage control surgery has been applied in the case of polytraumatized or resolved patients, the primary causes that induced the ACS are: The abdomen should preferably be left open, in peritoniostomy, using a temporary closure technique (Fig. 15.4). The requirements of any temporary abdominal closure technique are sufficient to provide decompression of the abdominal fascia. The optimal temporary abdominal closure should not harm the fascia, aponeurosis, or skin and should facilitate the gradual approach of the skin. The detailed discussion on the management of peritoneostomy is not part of the scope of this chapter; however, it is worth

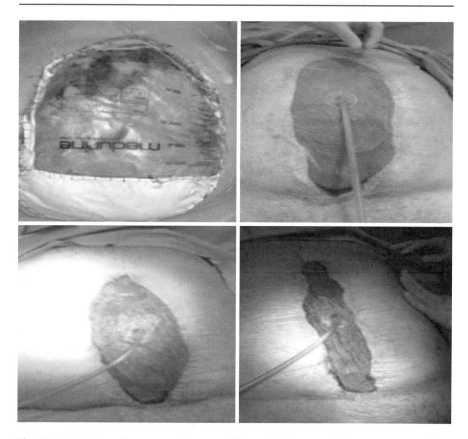

Fig. 15.4 Evolution of temporary closure technique with subatmospheric pressure therapy in a case of peritonitis (from authors library)

emphasizing that the techniques available for the maintenance of the open abdomen are important prevention strategies for ACS, however it has significant morbidity and mortality [17–20].

Recent publications showed that early surgical indication for the use of ACS resulted in about 80% fewer complications, including infections, sepsis, fistulas, and abscesses [19–22]. Percutaneous drainage of peritoneal fluid is an attractive and well-documented option in burn patients and in pediatric literature. This method can work in the presence of ascites for example; however, it is very unlikely to be efficient in the control of IAH/ACS of patients undergoing exploratory laparotomy, mainly traumatized undergoing damage control surgery where ACS is caused by intestinal edema, compresses used in abdominal packing, residual fluid, and clots22. Secondly, when the damage control technique is used, the patient presents with multiple intra-abdominal injuries and the presence of ACS on the first postoperative day means more likely re-bleeding and the percutaneous drainage of the abdomen clearly does not solve the problem. Recurrence of bleeding, obviously, requires reevaluation of abdominal hemostasis, with decompression and exploratory laparotomy [19–22]. Percutaneous drainage of the abdomen can be a valuable tool for a select group of patients where primary ACS develops during the non-operative treatment of isolated lesions in solid abdominal organs (liver and spleen). Another drainage option for patients who have an intra-abdominal hematoma retained by massive visceral trauma, mainly liver and who are in IAH refractory to clinical measures and in progressive evolution for ACS is videolaparoscopy, with washing and aspiration of the remaining content of the hematoma and revision of the cavity. Unfortunately, there is still no clear and concrete evidence of the indications of this technique; however, our service as well as other specialized services are made of this procedure as a useful tool, in these determined cases.

With regard to the treatment of the IAH/ACS, we then separate six steps that are especially important to be memorized:

1. Evacuate intraluminal intestinal contents.
2. Empty abdominal and/or retroperitoneal extracellular contents.
3. Improve abdominal compliance (for example: the use of neuromuscular blockers.
4. Optimize fluid management (balanced resuscitation/vasopressor).
5. Optimize tissue perfusion.
6. Indicate early surgical intervention.

15.7   Final Considerations and Conclusion

Abdominal compartment syndrome is a potentially lethal condition caused by any event that produces an increase in intra-abdominal pressure and causes a decrease in abdominal perfusion pressure, inducing ischemia and organ dysfunction. Its pathophysiological effects are wide and predispose to patients undergoing multiple organ failure if no urgent action is deliberate. Hemodynamic, renal, respiratory, and neurological abnormalities are common findings. Early decompressive laparotomy reduces the morbidity and mortality of patients affected by this serious condition and is the treatment of choice in cases refractory to clinical treatment.

The presence of abdominal compartment syndrome reflects the progressive evolution of intra-abdominal hypertension without adequate medical intervention. The World Society of the Abdominal Compartment classified the intra-abdominal hypertension into four grades and determined guidelines for the diagnosis and management of this clinical-surgical complication. As a consequence of the creation of the World Society of the Abdominal Compartment and the guidelines and protocols developed by more doctors and health professionals, they were exposed to the informative and educational content and can now perceive with more attention, the presence of the intra-abdominal hypertension or abdominal compartment syndrome.

References

1. Carr JA. Abdominal compartment syndrome: a decade of progress. J Am Coll Surg. 2013;216(1):135–46.
2. Kirkpatrick AW, Sugrue M, McKee JL, Pereira BM, Roberts DJ, De Waele JJ, Leppaniemi A, et al. Update from the Abdominal Compartment Society (WSACS) on intra-abdominal

hypertension and abdominal compartment syndrome: past, present, and future beyond Banff 2017. Anaesthesiol Intensive Ther. 2017;49(2):83–7.

3. Kirkpatrick AW, Roberts DJ, De Waele J, Jaeschke R, Malbrain ML, De Keulenaer B, et al. Intra-abdominal hypertension and the abdominal compartment syndrome: updated consensus definitions and clinical practice guidelines from the World Society of the Abdominal Compartment Syndrome. Intensive Care Med. 2013 Jul;39(7):1190–206.

4. World Society of the Abdominal Compartment Syndrome. Disponível em: http://www.wsacs.org/.

5. Sugrue M, Buhkari Y. Intra-abdominal pressure and abdominal compartment syndrome in acute general surgery. World J Surg. 2009;33(6):1123–7.

6. Ameloot K, Gillebert C, Desie N, Malbrain ML. Hypoperfusion, shock states, and abdominal compartment syndrome (ACS). Surg Clin North Am. 2012;92(2):207–20, vii.

7. Kirkpatrick AW, De Waele JJ, De Laet I, De Keulenaer BL, D'Amours S, Bjorck M, et al. WSACS—The Abdominal Compartment Society. A Society dedicated to the study of the physiology and pathophysiology of the abdominal compartment and its interactions with all organ systems. Anaesthesiol Intensive Ther. 2015;47(3):191–4.

8. Wise R, Roberts DJ, Vandervelden S, Debergh D, De Waele JJ, De Laet I, et al. Awareness and knowledge of intra-abdominal hypertension and abdominal compartment syndrome: results of an international survey. Anaesthesiol Intensive Ther. 2015;47(1):14–29.

9. Struck MF, Illert T, Schmidt T, Reichelt B, Steen M. Secondary abdominal compartment syndrome in patients with toxic epidermal necrolysis. Burns. 2012;38(4):562–7.

10. Duchesne JC, Howell MP, Eriksen C, Wahl GM, Rennie KV, Hastings PE, et al. Linea alba fasciotomy: a novel alternative in trauma patients with secondary abdominal compartment syndrome. Am Surg. 2010;76(3):312–6.

11. Cheatham ML, De Waele J, Kirkpatrick A, Sugrue M, Malbrain ML, Ivatury RR, et al. Criteria for a diagnosis of abdominal compartment syndrome. Can J Surg. 2009;52(4):315–6.

12. Luckianow GM, Ellis M, Governale D, Kaplan LJ. Abdominal compartment syndrome: risk factors, diagnosis, and current therapy. Crit Care Res Pract. 2012;2012:908169.

13. Harrell BR, Melander S. Identifying the association among risk factors and mortality in trauma patients with intra-abdominal hypertension and abdominal compartment syndrome. J Trauma Nurs. 2012;19(3):182–9.

14. Balogh ZJ, Leppaniemi A. Patient populations at risk for intra-abdominal hypertension and abdominal compartment syndrome. Am Surg. 2011;77 Suppl 1:S12–6.

15. Pereira BM, Pereira RG, Wise R, Sugrue G, Zakrison TL, Dorigatti AE, Fiorelli RK, Malbrain MLNG. The role of point-of-care ultrasound in intra-abdominal hypertension management. Anaesthesiol Intensive Ther. 2017;49(5):373–81.

16. Sugrue G, Malbrain MLNG, Pereira B, Wise R, Sugrue M. Modern imaging techniques in intra-abdominal hypertension and abdominal compartment syndrome: a bench to bedside overview. Anaesthesiol Intensive Ther. 2018;50(3):234–42.

17. Papavramidis TS, Marinis AD, Pliakos I, Kesisoglou I, Papavramidou N. Abdominal compartment syndrome—intra-abdominal hypertension: defining, diagnosing, and managing. J Emerg Trauma Shock. 2011;4(2):279–91.

18. Anand RJ, Ivatury RR. Surgical management of intra-abdominal hypertension and abdominal compartment syndrome. Am Surg. 2011;77 Suppl 1:S42–5.

19. Cheatham ML. Nonoperative management of intraabdominal hypertension and abdominal compartment syndrome. World J Surg. 2009;33(6):1116–22.

20. Cheatham ML, Safcsak K. Is the evolving management of intra-abdominal hypertension and abdominal compartment syndrome improving survival? Crit Care Med. 2010;38(2):402–7.

21. Balogh ZJ, Malbrain M. Resuscitation in intra-abdominal hypertension and abdominal compartment syndrome. Am Surg. 2011;77 Suppl 1:S31–3.

22. Rizoli S, Mamtani A, Scarpelini S, Kirkpatrick AW. Abdominal compartment syndrome in trauma resuscitation. Curr Opin Anaesthesiol. 2010;23(2):251–7.

Part II

Key Performance Indicators

Cholecystitis

16

Luca Ansaloni, Louise Flanagan, and Michael Sugrue

Title: The hospital report all patients admitted to the surgical service with acute cholecystitis and cholangitis

Description	No. of patients with acute calculous cholecystitis (ACC) and cholangitis admitted
Rationale	Provides an estimate of overall number requiring care
Target	All patients
KPI reporting	6 monthly
Data sources	EGS registry

Title: The hospital report its laparoscopic conversion rate in cholecystectomy

Description	Percentage of patients with ACC operated on with laparoscopy with conversion to open surgery
Rationale	Provides an estimate of the level of patient complexity and surgical care
Target	All patients undergoing surgery for ACC

L. Ansaloni (✉)
Unit of General and Emergency Surgery, Bufalini Hospital of Cesena, AUSL Romagna, Cesena, Forlì-Cesena, Italy
e-mail: luca.ansaloni@auslromagna.it

L. Flanagan
Department of Surgery, EU INTERREG Emergency Surgery Outcomes Advancement Project (eSOAP), Letterkenny University Hospital, Letterkenny, Co. Donegal, Ireland
e-mail: Louise.Flanagan@hse.ie

M. Sugrue
Letterkenny University Hospital and University Hospital Galway, Letterkenny, Donegal, Ireland

EU INTERREG Emergency Surgery Outcomes Advancement Project (eSOAP), Letterkenny University Hospital, Letterkenny, Donegal, Ireland

| KPI reporting | 6 monthly |
| Data sources | EGS registry |

Title: The hospital report its incomplete laparoscopic rate in cholecystectomy

Description	Percentage of patients with ACC operated where the gallbladder is not removed, but there is not a conversion to open
Rationale	Provides an estimate of the level of patient complexity and surgical care and indicates the number undergoing either subtotal cholecystectomy, laparoscopic cholecystostomy or bail out procedure
Target	All patients undergoing laparoscopic surgery
KPI reporting	6 monthly
Data sources	EGS registry

Title: Timing of surgery in ACC

Description	Percentage of patients with ACC operated on with operation performed within first 6 days post-admission
Rationale	Appropriate timing for operative management of ACC is within 6 days post-admission in most patients
Target	>90% of patients with ACC are operated within 6 days post-admission
KPI reporting	6 monthly
Data sources	EGS registry

Title: Index admission surgery is undertaken in patients presenting with ACC

Description	Patients admitted with ACC get surgery on their first admission
Rationale	Early surgery is indicated in most patients. A number of patients will decline or be unfit for surgery
Target	80% of patients admitted with ACC get surgery on their first admission
KPI reporting	6 monthly
Data sources	EGS registry

Title: Re-admission following either cholecystectomy, cholecystostomy or ERCP

Description	Any patient re-admitted following a biliary intervention within 90 days
Rationale	Provide an understanding of the outcome for the patient
Target	<5% of patients are re-admitted
KPI reporting	6 monthly
Data sources	EGS registry

Title: Unplanned re-admission following non-operative approach to initial ACC

Description	Any patient re-admitted following non-operative management within 90 days of their admission
Rationale	Capture the outcome for the patient
Target	<5% of patients are re-admitted
KPI reporting	6 monthly
Data sources	EGS registry

Pancreatitis

17

Ari Leppaniemi

17.1 Pancreatitis KPI 1

Title: Need for Intensive Care Unit treatment

Description	Percentage of patients with acute pancreatitis treated in the ICU
Rationale	Patients with organ failures should be admitted early to the ICU.
Target	>90% of patients admitted for acute pancreatitis with early organ dysfunction (defined as SOFA score >3 within the first 24 h) within 24 h post-admission
KPI collection frequency	Semi-annually
KPI reporting frequency	Semi-annually
KPI calculation	Numerator divided by denominator expressed as a percentage Numerator: Number of patients with acute pancreatitis and early organ dysfunction admitted to the ICU Denominator: Number of all patients with acute pancreatitis and early organ dysfunction admitted to the hospital
Reporting aggregation	National, regional, LHO area, hospital, age, gender
Data sources	Administrative data, Medical records

A. Leppaniemi (✉)
Abdominal Center, Helsinki University Hospital, Helsinki, Finland
e-mail: Ari.Leppaniemi@hus.fi

© World Society of Emergency Surgery and Donegal Clinical and Research Academy 2020   133
M. Sugrue et al. (eds.), *Resources for Optimal Care of Emergency Surgery*,
Hot Topics in Acute Care Surgery and Trauma,
https://doi.org/10.1007/978-3-030-49363-9_17

17.2   Pancreatitis KPI 2

Title: Prevention of the need for surgical decompression for Abdominal Compartment Syndrome (ACS)

Description	Percentage of patients with acute pancreatitis with measured intra-abdominal pressure (IAP) >20 mmHg within first 3 days post-admission
Rationale	Appropriate non-operative management on intra-abdominal hypertension (IAH) (decreasing the volume of intra-abdominal content including percutaneous drainage of ascites, improving abdominal wall compliance, removing excess fluid with negative fluid balance, etc.) should be able to prevent the development of ACS in most patients.
Target	>70% of patients with early IAH should avoid progression to ACS.
KPI collection frequency	Semi-annually
KPI reporting frequency	Semi-annually
KPI calculation	Numerator divided by denominator expressed as a percentage Numerator: Number of patients with acute pancreatitis and early IAH avoiding decompressive surgery Denominator: Number of all patients with acute pancreatitis and early IAH
Reporting aggregation	National, regional, LHO area, hospital, age, gender
Data sources	Administrative data, Medical records

17.3   Pancreatitis KPI 3

Title: Delayed fascial closure (DFC) rate after decompressive laparostomy for ACS

Description	Percentage of patients with acute pancreatitis achieving DFC after decompressive laparostomy
Rationale	Successful temporary abdominal closure (TAC) techniques results in high DFC.
Target	>90% of patients undergoing decompressive laparostomy achieving DFC
KPI collection frequency	Semi-annually
KPI reporting frequency	Semi-annually
KPI calculation	Numerator divided by denominator expressed as a percentage Numerator: Number of patients with acute pancreatitis undergoing decompressive surgery achieving DFC Denominator: Number of all patients with acute pancreatitis undergoing decompressive laparostomy and some form of TAC
Reporting aggregation	National, regional, LHO area, hospital, age, gender
Data sources	Administrative data, Medical records

17.4 Pancreatitis KPI 4

Title: Benefit of surgical necrosectomy

Description	Percentage of patients with infected pancreatic necrosis getting better after surgical necrosectomy (regardless of technique used)
Rationale	Necrosectomy for infected pancreatic necrosis, when performed at the right time (>4 weeks post-admission, walled-off necrosis—WON) and for appropriate indications should result in improved organ function and eventually outcome.
Target	>80% of patients undergoing surgical necrosectomy should have decrease of SOFA score of >3 points by 5th postoperative day.
KPI collection frequency	Semi-annually
KPI reporting frequency	Semi-annually
KPI calculation	Numerator divided by denominator expressed as a percentage Numerator: Number of patients with infected necrosis treated with surgical necrosectomy improving their SOFA score by >3 points by 5th postoperative day Denominator: Number of all patients with infected necrosis treated with surgical necrosectomy
Reporting aggregation	National, regional, LHO area, hospital, age, gender
Data sources	Administrative data, Medical records

17.5 Pancreatitis KPI 5

Title: Hospital mortality in severe acute pancreatitis

Description	Percentage of patients with severe acute pancreatitis dying during the initial hospital stay period
Rationale	At least 80% of patients with severe acute pancreatitis (definition: acute pancreatitis with infected necrosis and/or persistent organ failure with SOFA score >2 of renal, respiratory, or cardiovascular organ systems) should survive the initial hospitalization period.
Target	>80% of patients with severe acute pancreatitis
KPI collection frequency	Semi-annually
KPI reporting frequency	Semi-annually
KPI calculation	Numerator divided by denominator expressed as a percentage Numerator: Number of patients with severe acute pancreatitis surviving the initial hospital treatment period Denominator: Number of all patients with severe acute pancreatitis admitted
Reporting aggregation	National, regional, LHO area, hospital, age, gender
Data sources	Administrative data, Medical records

Further Reading

Banks PA, Bollen TL, Dervenis C, Gooszen HG, Johnson CD, Sarr MG, et al. Classification of acute pancreatitis—2012: revision of the Atlanta classification and definitions by international consensus. Gut. 2013;62:102–11.

Besselink MG, Van Santvoort HC, Boermeester MA, Nieuweohuijs VB, Van Goor H, Dejong CHC, et al. Timing and impact of infections in acute pancreatitis. Br J Surg. 2009;96:267–73.

Halonen KI, Pettilä V, Leppäniemi AK, Kemppainen EA, Puolakkainen PA, Haapiainen RK. Multiple organ dysfunction associated with severe acute pancreatitis. Crit Care Med. 2002;30:1274–9.

Husu HL, Leppäniemi AK, Lehtonen TM, Puolakkainen PA, Mentula PJ. Short- and long-term survival after severe acute pancreatitis: a retrospective 17 years' cohort study from a single center. J Crit Care. 2019;53:81–6.

Leppäniemi AK. Laparostomy: why and when? Crit Care. 2010;14:216.

Leppäniemi A, Tolonen M, Tarasconi A, Segovia-Lohse H, Gamberini E, Kirkpatrick AW, et al. WSES guidelines for the management of severe acute pancreatitis. World J Emerg Surg. 2019;14:27. https://doi.org/10.1186/s13017-019-0247-0.

Mentula P, Hienonen P, Kemppainen E, Puolakkainen P, Leppäniemi A. Surgical decompression for abdominal compartment syndrome in severe acute pancreatitis. Arch Surg. 2010;145:764–9.

van Santvoort HC, Besselink MG, Bakker OJ, Hofker HS, Boermeester MA, Dejong CH, et al. A step-up approach or open necrosectomy for necrotizing pancreatitis. N Engl J Med. 2010;362:1491–502.

Upper GI Bleed

18

Chris Steele

Patients who are admitted to hospital with upper GI who are hypotensive (<100 mmHg) for more than 30 min need to be admitted to a high dependency unit

Description	Unstable upper GI bleeding patients are admitted to a high dependency unit.
Rationale	Patients who are unstable with upper GI bleeding have a worse outcome and need close monitoring to tailor treatment modalities, in particular serial Hb and frequent vital sign monitoring.
Target	80% of patients admitted with an unstable upper GI bleed (BP < 100 mmHg) should be in a HDU within 2 hours of arrival in Emergency Department.
KPI reporting	6 monthly
Data sources	EGS registry

Patients with blood per rectum have their anticoagulants stopped on admission and are not charted for heparins in the first 12 hours post admission

Description	Patients with blood per rectum have their anticoagulants stopped on admission and are not charted for heparins in the first 12 hours post admission. This would include antiplatelet agents and warfarin.
Rationale	Patients who present with blood per rectum may be on anticoagulants, usually for atrial fibrillation. They may have a recent stent or history of thromboembolic phenomenon. Failure to stop these medications at least for the first few hours of admission could result in more significant hemorrhage.
Target	95% of patients admitted for blood per rectum have their anticoagulants stopped.
KPI reporting	6 monthly
Data sources	EGS registry

C. Steele (✉)
Letterkenny University Hospital, Letterkenny, Co. Donegal, Ireland
e-mail: Chris.Steele@hse.ie

© World Society of Emergency Surgery and Donegal Clinical and Research Academy 2020   137
M. Sugrue et al. (eds.), *Resources for Optimal Care of Emergency Surgery*,
Hot Topics in Acute Care Surgery and Trauma,
https://doi.org/10.1007/978-3-030-49363-9_18

Bowel Obstruction

19

Randal Parlour, Manvydas Varzgalis, and Brendan Skelly

19.1 Small Bowel Obstruction

Title: Pathway for SBO management

Description	Patients admitted with SBO should be enrolled in a hospital SBO pathway.
Rationale	Pathways including use of gastrografin improve outcome.
Target	>90%
KPI reporting	6 monthly
Data sources	EGS registry

R. Parlour (✉)
EU INTERREG Emergency Surgery Outcomes Advancement Project (eSOAP),
Letterkenny University Hospital, Letterkenny, Co. Donegal, Ireland

Ulster University, Derry, Northern Ireland, UK
e-mail: Randal.Parlour@hse.ie

M. Varzgalis
Letterekenny University Hospital, Letterkenny, Co. Donegal, Ireland
e-mail: Manvydas.Varzgalis1@hse.ie

B. Skelly
EU INTERREG Emergency Surgery Outcomes Advancement Project (eSOAP),
Letterkenny University Hospital, Letterkenny, Co. Donegal, Ireland

Department of Surgery, Altnagelvin Hospital, Derry, Northern Ireland, UK
e-mail: brendan.skelly@westerntrust.hscni.net

© World Society of Emergency Surgery and Donegal Clinical and Research Academy 2020   139
M. Sugrue et al. (eds.), *Resources for Optimal Care of Emergency Surgery*,
Hot Topics in Acute Care Surgery and Trauma,
https://doi.org/10.1007/978-3-030-49363-9_19

Title: Suspected SBO—CT scan

Description	New patients over the age of 35 years presenting with suspected SBO should undergo abdominal CT with IV and oral contrast (unless specific contraindications).
Rationale	To confirm the diagnosis and to differentiate between other acute abdominal/pelvic pathologies, for surgery preparedness and strategy
Target	>90%
KPI reporting	6 monthly
Data sources	EGS registry

Title: Timing of surgery and outcome

Description	The small bowel resection rate in those undergoing surgery should be less than 30%.
Rationale	Perforation following ischaemia will increase mortality.
Target	<30%
KPI reporting	6 monthly
Data sources	EGS registry

19.2 Large Bowel Obstruction

Title: Patients with large bowel obstruction have underlying diagnosis made within 24 h of presentation.

Description	Ensure effective prompt clinical treatment, and prevention of perforation
Rationale	To ensure prompt clinical treatment avoid complications from bowel perforations and ischaemia.
Target	90% patients with LBO diagnosis
KPI reporting	6 monthly
Data sources	EGS registry

Title: Leak rate in patients under primary anastomosis is less than 10%

Description	Understanding the clinical outcomes of emergency surgery is essential in improving outcome.
Rationale	Identification of leak rate beyond 10% for acute surgery would suggest need for remedial action.
Target	Leak rate < 10% patients with LBO diagnosis under anastomosis during their care
KPI reporting	6 monthly
Data sources	EGS registry

Perforated Gastroduodenal Ulcer (PGDU)

20

Kjetil Soreide

20.1 Aim

To outline key standards and develop measurement KPIs for emergency surgery for perforated gastroduodenal ulcers.

20.2 Definition and Background

Perforated gastroduodenal ulcers (PGDU) refer to a spontaneous perforation of the gastric or duodenal wall associated with free air (on imaging), localized or generalized peritonitis with or without associated sepsis syndrome [1]. The condition is associated with increased mortality with delay to diagnosis, delay to surgery, in the elderly and in the comorbid patients.

While peptic ulcer incidence and associated complications (bleeding and obstruction) have dropped over the past decades, the perforation rate has been fairly consistent. The mortality rate in perforated gastroduodenal ulcers (PGDU) remains high (from 10% to 30%), with notable geographic differences [2]. The latter is due to demographic differences between regions, with duodenal perforations in young men being predominant in low- and middle-income countries, while a shift towards gastric location in elderly and slight female predominance is seen in high-income countries. Outcome is associated with age, presence of comorbidity and strongly linked to delay in diagnosis and treatment [2]. CT is the preferred modality for imaging due to the superior accuracy and ability to detect differentials [3]. Early resuscitation and antibiotics should be emphasized and prompt surgery performed [4–6]. Surgical repair can be done as open or laparoscopic, with no differences in major outcomes [7]. Non-operative management may

K. Soreide (✉)
Department of Gastrointestinal Surgery, Stavanger University Hospital, Stavanger, Norway

Department of Clinical Medicine, University of Bergen, Bergen, Norway

© World Society of Emergency Surgery and Donegal Clinical and Research Academy 2020   141
M. Sugrue et al. (eds.), *Resources for Optimal Care of Emergency Surgery*,
Hot Topics in Acute Care Surgery and Trauma,
https://doi.org/10.1007/978-3-030-49363-9_20

be discussed in select patients, but has low-grade evidence support and may have a high failure rate in elderly [1]. Post-op monitoring for organ failure, appropriate organ support and preferable high-dependency unit surveillance or ICU care should be considered. Reoperation rates are reported at 15–20% and most often due to leaks [8], and should be kept to a lowest possible rate. In patients not improving after surgery, a persistent leak or intra-abdominal collection should be aggressively diagnosed and managed, either percutaneously (collections) or by reoperation (leaks).

20.3   PGDU KPI 1

Title: Timing of surgery

Description	Percentage of patients with PDGU operated on with operation performed within first 6 h of diagnosis (e.g. clinical and/or imaging)
Rationale	Appropriate timing for operative management of PDGU is within 6 h in most patients.
Target	>90% of patients with PDGU are operated within 6 hours post-admission.
KPI collection frequency	Semi-annually
KPI reporting frequency	Semi-annually
KPI calculation	Numerator divided by denominator expressed as a percentage Numerator: Number of patients with PDGU operated within 6 h after diagnosis post-admission Denominator: Number of all patients with PDGU operated
Reporting aggregation	National, regional, LHO area, hospital, age, gender
Data sources	Administrative data, Medical records

20.4   PGDU KPI 2

Title: Patients admitted with suspected PDGU should have an abdominal CT done within 4 h of admission (within time since suspected diagnosis if in-house)

Description	Performance of abdominal CT
Rationale	Timely investigation to obtain the diagnosis of PDGU is important. Patients presenting with symptoms suggestive of PDGU should be prioritized to have the CT as an emergency priority. They may then be potentially scheduled for surgery the following day on the emergency list.
Target	80% of patients presenting to Emergency Department should have an abdominal CT within 4 h
KPI collection frequency	Monthly
KPI reporting frequency	Monthly
KPI calculation	Numerator divided by denominator expressed as a percentage Numerator: Number of emergency surgery patients admitted with PDGU, having presented to Emergency department (or similar location) who have an abdominal CT Denominator: Number of emergency surgery patients admitted with PDGU having presented to Emergency department (or similar location) prior to 1600 (daytime)
Reporting aggregation	Hospital 1
Data sources	Emergency Surgery Database, radiology reporting systems

20.5   PGDU KPI 3

Title: Reporting of the outcomes from surgery

Description	Documented reported outcome from surgery
Rationale	The incidence of complication needs to be reported from hospitals to maintain quality and improve outcome.
Target	100% of patients undergoing PDGU repair are entered into a hospital wide registry with data retrievable for intra-abdominal collections, leaks, reoperation, organ failure/support.
KPI collection frequency	6 monthly
KPI reporting frequency	6 monthly
KPI calculation	Numerator divided by denominator expressed as a percentage
	Numerator: Reporting of the outcomes from surgery
	Denominator: 6 months
Reporting aggregation	Hospital
Data sources	Emergency Surgery Database, patients notes

20.6   PGDU KPI 4

Title: Hospital mortality in PDGU; overall mortality at 90 days

Description	Percentage of patients with PDGU dying during the first 30 days period; overall mortality at 90 days
Rationale	At least 85% patients with PDGU should survive the initial 30 days period
Target	>85% of patients with PDGU surviving the initial 30 days period (age- and gender-dependent outcome)
KPI collection frequency	Semi-annually
KPI reporting frequency	Semi-annually
KPI calculation	Numerator divided by denominator expressed as a percentage
	Numerator: Number of patients with PDGU surviving the initial 30 days period
	Denominator: Number of all patients with PDGU admitted
Reporting aggregation	National, regional, LHO area, hospital, age, gender
Data sources	Administrative data, Medical records

20.7   PGDU KPI 5

Title: Laparoscopic surgery

Description	Percentage of patients with PDGU operated on with laparoscopic initial attempt
Rationale	Initial laparoscopic attempt in PDGU surgery is appropriate.
Target	50–80% of patients with PDGU undergoing surgery receive an initial laparoscopic approach.
KPI collection frequency	Semi-annually
KPI reporting frequency	Semi-annually
KPI calculation	Numerator divided by denominator expressed as a percentage Numerator: Number of patients with PDGU undergoing surgery receiving initial laparoscopic approach Denominator: Number of all patients with PDGU undergoing surgery
Reporting aggregation	National, regional, LHO area, hospital, age, gender

References

1. Søreide K, Thorsen K, Harrison EM, et al. Perforated peptic ulcer. Lancet. 2015;386:1288–98.
2. Søreide K, Thorsen K, Soreide JA. Clinical patterns of presentation and attenuated inflammatory response in octo- and nonagenarians with perforated gastroduodenal ulcers. Surgery. 2016;160:341–9.
3. Thorsen K, Glomsaker TB, von Meer A, et al. Trends in diagnosis and surgical management of patients with perforated peptic ulcer. J Gastrointest Surg. 2011;15:1329–35.
4. Soreide K, Thorsen K, Soreide JA. Strategies to improve the outcome of emergency surgery for perforated peptic ulcer. Br J Surg. 2014;101:e51–64.
5. Moller MH, Larsson HJ, Rosenstock S, et al. Quality-of-care initiative in patients treated surgically for perforated peptic ulcer. Br J Surg. 2013;100:543–52.
6. Buck DL, Vester-Andersen M, Moller MH. Surgical delay is a critical determinant of survival in perforated peptic ulcer. Br J Surg. 2013;100:1045–9.
7. Cirocchi R, Soreide K, Di Saverio S, et al. Meta-analysis of perioperative outcomes of acute laparoscopic versus open repair of perforated gastroduodenal ulcers. J Trauma Acute Care Surg. 2018;85:417–25.
8. Wilhelmsen M, Moller MH, Rosenstock S. Surgical complications after open and laparoscopic surgery for perforated peptic ulcer in a nationwide cohort. Br J Surg. 2015;102:382–7.

Acute Diverticulitis (AD): Management Phase

21

Marja Boermeester

21.1 Acute Diverticulitis KPI 1

Title: Diagnosis of complicated AD

Description	Optimising outcome
Rationale	The mortality rate among patients with Hinchey 3 or 4 should be less than current international results.
Target	>95% of patients with Hinchey 3 or 4 AD who had emergency surgery is operated only after preoperative imaging (US and/or CT).
KPI collection frequency	Quarterly
KPI reporting frequency	Quarterly
KPI calculation	Numerator divided by denominator expressed as a percentage
	Numerator: Number of patients with preoperative US and/or CT imaging in patient group with Hinchey 3 or 4 AD who had emergency surgery
	Denominator: Total number of patients with Hinchey 3 or 4 AD who had emergency
Reporting aggregation	Hospital, Hospital Group
Data sources	Patient charts, hospital discharge data, emergency surgery database

M. Boermeester (✉)
Department of Surgery, Amsterdam UMC, location AMC, Amsterdam, The Netherlands
e-mail: m.a.boermeester@amsterdamumc.nl

© World Society of Emergency Surgery and Donegal Clinical and Research Academy 2020   145
M. Sugrue et al. (eds.), *Resources for Optimal Care of Emergency Surgery*,
Hot Topics in Acute Care Surgery and Trauma,
https://doi.org/10.1007/978-3-030-49363-9_21

21.2 Acute Diverticulitis KPI 2

Title: Mortality rate associated with AD

Description	Optimising outcome
Rationale	The mortality rate among patients with Hinchey 3 or 4 should be less than current international results.
Target	Mortality rate < 10% of patients with peritonitis due to Hinchey 3 or 4 AD
KPI collection frequency	Quarterly
KPI reporting frequency	Quarterly
KPI calculation	Numerator divided by denominator expressed as a percentage Numerator: Number of deaths in patient group with Hinchey 3 or 4 AD Denominator: Total number of patients with Hinchey 3 or 4 AD
Reporting aggregation	Hospital, Hospital Group
Data sources	Patient charts, hospital discharge data, emergency surgery database

21.3 Acute Diverticulitis KPI 3

Title: Timely antibiotic administration in complicated acute diverticulitis

Description	Self-explanatory
Rationale	To ensure minimum interval between imaging diagnosis of acute complicated diverticulitis and institution of appropriate antibiotic. Early sepsis control will ensure greater survival. Patients with uncomplicated diverticulitis do not need antibiotics routinely.
Target	All patients with complicated diverticulitis and either localised or generalised peritonitis have timely antibiotic administration.
KPI collection frequency	Quarterly
KPI reporting frequency	Quarterly
KPI calculation	Numerator divided by denominator expressed as a percentage Numerator: Number of patients with imaging confirmed complicated acute diverticulitis (Hinchey II, III or IV) who had empiric antibiotic management initiated within 1 h of imaging diagnosis Denominator: Total number of patients with imaging confirmed complicated acute diverticulitis
Reporting aggregation	Hospital, Hospital Group
Data sources	EGS Registry

21.4   Acute Diverticulitis KPI 4

Title: Bacteriological identification of flora in abscess or peritoneal cavity

Description	Optimising a targeted antibiotic regime to enhance bacterial kills and reduce Clostridium difficile and antimicrobial resistance.
Rationale	To ensure appropriate targeted antibiotic treatment instituted, to avoid the emergence of antibiotic resistance and to promote antibiotic stewardship
Target	All patients with acute diverticulitis undergoing radiological or surgical drainage or surgical resection have a culture sample taken
KPI collection frequency	Quarterly
KPI reporting frequency	Quarterly
KPI calculation	Numerator divided by denominator expressed as a percentage Numerator: Number of patients with diverticulitis undergoing radiological or surgical drainage or surgical resection, where samples were forwarded for cultures and sensitivity pattern Denominator: Total number of patients with diverticulitis undergoing radiological or surgical drainage or surgical resection
Reporting aggregation	Hospital, Hospital Group
Deta sources	Patient charts, HIPE, diverticular disease database if maintained, microbiology laboratory reports

21.5   Acute Diverticulitis KPI 5a

Title: Follow-up colonoscopy post discharge in patients with diagnosis of acute diverticulitis and persistent complaints

Description	Self-explanatory
Rationale	To out rule the presence of an underlying colon cancer. Uncomplicated transient AD is not associated with colon cancer. Complicated or persistent AD may obscure the diagnosis of underlying colon cancer.
Target	>95% of patients with diagnosis of acute diverticulitis with persistent complaints for more than 1 month undergo colonoscopy within 3 months after diagnosis.
KPI collection frequency	Quarterly
KPI reporting frequency	Quarterly
KPI calculation	Numerator divided by denominator expressed as a percentage Numerator: All patients newly diagnosed with acute diverticulitis and persistent complaints for more than 1 month having colonoscopy within 3 months following index admission diagnosis Denominator: Total number of patients newly diagnosed with acute diverticulitis and persistent complaints for more than 1 month
Reporting aggregation	Hospital, Hospital Group
Data sources	Patient charts, hospital discharge data, emergency surgery database

21.6   Acute Diverticulitis KPI 5b

Title: Follow-up colonoscopy post discharge in patients with diagnosis of acute diverticulitis with abscess formation

Description	Self-explanatory
Rationale	To out rule the presence of an underlying colon cancer
Target	>95% of patients with diagnosis of acute diverticulitis with abscess formation (irrespective of the size) undergo colonoscopy within 3 months after diagnosis.
KPI collection frequency	Quarterly
KPI reporting frequency	Quarterly
KPI calculation	Numerator divided by denominator expressed as a percentage Numerator: All patients newly diagnosed with acute diverticulitis and abscess formation having colonoscopy within 3 months following index admission diagnosis Denominator: Total number of patients newly diagnosed with acute diverticulitis and abscess formation
Reporting aggregation	Hospital, Hospital Group
Data sources	Patient charts, hospital discharge data, emergency surgery database

21.7   Acute Diverticulitis KPI 6

Title: BhCG performed in female patients of childbearing age presenting with suspected AD

Description	BhCG
Rationale	To out rule pregnancy especially left-sided ectopic
Target	All female patients of childbearing age presenting with suspected AD have BhCG performed.
KPI collection frequency	Quarterly
KPI reporting frequency	Quarterly
KPI calculation	Numerator divided by denominator expressed as a percentage Numerator: Number of female patients of childbearing age presenting with suspected AD who had a BhCG performed at the emergency department Denominator: Total number of female patients of childbearing age presenting with suspected AD
Reporting aggregation	Hospital, Hospital Group
Data sources	EGS registry

Abdominal Vascular Emergencies

22

Scott Thomas

22.1 Non-traumatic Abdominal Vascular Emergencies

22.1.1 Abdominal Vascular Emergencies KPI 1

Title: Patients admitted with suspected non-traumatic abdominal vascular emergencies (NTAVE)

Description	Timely performance of baseline laboratory tests including base deficit or lactic acid, and CT scan and/or angiography
Rationale	Timely investigation to obtain the diagnosis of NTAVE to determine if AAA, non-AAA, etiology of NTAVE is essential.
Target	100% of patients presenting to the Emergency Department with NTAVE
KPI collection frequency	Monthly
KPI reporting frequency	Monthly
KPI calculation	Numerator divided by denominator expressed as a percentage Numerator: Number of with patients timely performance of baseline laboratory tests including base deficit or lactic acid, and CT scan and/or angiography presenting to the Emergency Department with NTAVE Denominator: Number of patients presenting to the Emergency Department with NTAVE
Reporting aggregation	Hospital 1
Data sources	Emergency Surgery Database, Radiology Reporting Systems, Laboratory Reporting Systems, ICU, and Medical Unit Database

S. Thomas (✉)
General Surgery, Trauma Surgery, Beacon Medical Group Trauma and Surgical Services, South Bend, IN, USA
e-mail: sthomas@beaconhealthsystem.org

© World Society of Emergency Surgery and Donegal Clinical and Research Academy 2020   149
M. Sugrue et al. (eds.), *Resources for Optimal Care of Emergency Surgery*,
Hot Topics in Acute Care Surgery and Trauma,
https://doi.org/10.1007/978-3-030-49363-9_22

22.1.2 Abdominal Vascular Emergencies KPI 2

Title: Reporting of the outcomes from surgery

Description	Documented reported outcome from surgery (open or endovascular)
Rationale	The incidence of complications needs to be reported from hospitals to maintain quality and improve outcome.
Target	100% of patients undergoing NTAVE either open or EVAR are entered into a hospital wide registry with data retrievable for acute graft occlusion, bowel ischemia, endo leak, or death.
KPI collection frequency	6 months
KPI reporting frequency	6 months
KPI calculation	Numerator divided by denominator expressed as a percentage Numerator: Reporting of the outcomes from surgery Denominator: All patients in 6 months
Reporting aggregation	Hospital 1
Data sources	Emergency Surgery Database

22.1.3 Abdominal Vascular Emergencies KPI 3

Title: Reporting of the outcomes from supportive medical treatment

Description	Documented reported outcome from supportive medical treatment
Rationale	The incidence of complication needs to be reported from hospitals to maintain quality and improve outcomes.
Target	100% of patients undergoing medical treatment for NTAVE are entered into a hospital wide registry with data retrievable for AMI, SMA, SMV, vena cava, pelvic, iliac, portal venous thrombosis.
KPI collection frequency	6 months
KPI reporting frequency	6 months
KPI calculation	Numerator divided by denominator expressed as a percentage Numerator: Number of patients undergoing medical treatment for NTAVE are entered into a hospital wide registry with data retrievable for AMI, SMA, SMV, vena cava, pelvic, iliac, portal venous thrombosis Denominator: All patients medically treated for NTAVE over 6 months
Reporting aggregation	Hospital 1
Data sources	Emergency Surgery Database, ICU, and Medical Unit Database

22.2   Abdominal Aortic Aneurysms (AAA)

22.2.1 Abdominal Vascular Emergencies KPI 4

Title: Patients admitted with suspected AAA with hemodynamic instability should have US, FAST, and/or CT performed immediately

Description	Performance of US, FAST, and/or CT performed immediately
Rationale	Timely investigation to obtain the diagnosis of AAA is vital as it will result in death within 85–90% of rupture cases if not treated immediately.
Target	100% of patients presenting to Emergency Department with AAA
KPI collection frequency	Monthly
KPI reporting frequency	Monthly
KPI calculation	Numerator divided by denominator expressed as a percentage
	Numerator: Number of emergency surgery patients admitted with AAA who received US, FAST, and/or CT
	Denominator: Number of emergency surgery patients admitted with diagnosis of AAA.
Reporting aggregation	Hospital 1
Data sources	Emergency Surgery Database, Radiology Reporting Systems, Emergency Department Chart Review

22.2.2 Abdominal Vascular Emergencies KPI 5

Title: Patients admitted with hemodynamically unstable AAA need to be assessed by a consultant surgeon within 30 min of admission

Description	Documented consultant review
Rationale	Consultant surgeon input in patients with hemodynamically unstable AAA will optimize care and expedite investigation and surgery.
Target	100% of patients admitted with hemodynamically unstable AAA need to be assessed by a consultant surgeon within 30 min of admission.
KPI collection frequency	6 months
KPI reporting frequency	6 months
KPI calculation	Numerator divided by denominator expressed as a percentage
	Numerator: Patients admitted with hemodynamically unstable AAA need to be assessed by a consultant surgeon within 30 min of admission
	Denominator: Total patients admitted with hemodynamically unstable AAA
Reporting aggregation	Hospital 1
Data sources	Emergency Surgery Database

22.3   Non-Abdominal Aortic Aneurysms (Non-AAA)

22.3.1 Abdominal Vascular Emergencies KPI 6

Title: Patients admitted with non-AAA abdominal vascular emergencies will undergo radiologic vascular imaging, and treated with either stenting, endovascular thrombolysis, supportive medical care, or exploratory laparotomy (for detection of bowel viability, vascular pathology, or aneurysm repair).

Description	Patients should receive one of these diagnostic evaluations
Rationale	Detection of AMI, visceral aneurysm, iliac aneurysms, aortic dissection, spontaneous abdominal/retroperitoneal bleeding, SMA thrombosis/embolism, aortoenteric fistula, pelvic, iliac, vena cava thrombosis is essential for proper therapeutic decisions.
Target	100% of patients with non-AAA abdominal vascular emergencies should be evaluated with radiologic vascular imaging and treated with either stenting, endovascular thrombolysis, supportive medical care, or exploratory laparotomy (for bowel viability, vascular pathology, or aneurysm repair).
KPI collection frequency	6 months
KPI reporting frequency	6 months
KPI calculation	Numerator divided by denominator expressed as a percentage Numerator: Number of patients with non-AAA abdominal vascular emergencies should be evaluated with radiologic vascular imaging and treated with either stenting endovascular thrombolysis, supportive medical care, or exploratory laparotomy (for bowel viability, vascular pathology, or aneurysm repair) Denominator: Number of emergency surgery patients admitted with non-AAA abdominal vascular emergencies will undergo radiologic vascular imaging, and treated with either stenting, endovascular thrombolysis, supportive medical care, or exploratory laparotomy (for detection of bowel viability, vascular pathology, or aneurysm repair)
Reporting aggregation	Hospital 1
Data sources	Emergency Surgery Database, Radiology Database, Intensive Care and Medical Unit Database

Coagulation

23

Ernest E. Moore

KPI title: Patients requiring an emergent operation on warfarin therapy should have an international normalized ratio (INR) measured at the time of initial assessment

Description	INR measurement
Rationale	An emergent operation can be complicated with bleeding which may be accentuated due to warfarin therapy because of inadequate concentrations of clotting factors II, VII, IX, and X.
Target	100% of patients undergoing an emergent operation on warfarin therapy have a preoperative INR measured.
KPI collection frequency	Annually
KPI reporting frequency	Annually
KPI calculation	Numerator: number of patients undergoing an emergent operation on warfarin therapy who have a preoperative INR measured Denominator: number of patients undergoing an emergent operation on warfarin therapy
Reporting aggregation	Hospital 1
Data source(s)	Emergency surgery database ICU database

The original version of the book was revised: Affiliation of one of the editors, Ernest E. Moore, has been updated. The correction to the book is available at https://doi.org/10.1007/978-3-030-49363-9_26

E. E. Moore (✉)
Ernest E Moore Shock Trauma Center, Denver Health, Denver, CO, USA
e-mail: Ernest.Moore@dhha.org

© World Society of Emergency Surgery and Donegal Clinical and Research Academy 2020   153
M. Sugrue et al. (eds.), *Resources for Optimal Care of Emergency Surgery*,
Hot Topics in Acute Care Surgery and Trauma,
https://doi.org/10.1007/978-3-030-49363-9_23

Wound Care

24

Michael Sugrue

24.1 Wound Care

Emergency surgery patients under SSI surveillance

Description	Measurement of SSI and surgical site occurrence
Rationale	Optimising patient outcome through reduction in surgical site occurrence is crucial. Understanding the prevalence of SSI and SSO is vital to reducing complications and minimising cost. This translates to happier patients and families.
Target	90% of patients who undergo laparotomy are subject to SSI surveillance 3 monthly
KPI reporting	6 monthly
Data sources	EGS registry

24.2 Wound Care

A wound care bundle to include pre-operative, intra-operative, and post-operative key interventions KPI 50

Description	Documented compliance with wound care bundle.
Rationale	Wound infection can be markedly reduced by a collaborative approach in wound infection reduction.
Target	90% of emergency abdominal surgery has compliance with wound care bundle.
KPI reporting	6 monthly
Data sources	EGS registry

M. Sugrue (✉)
EU INTERREG Emergency Surgery Outcomes Advancement Project (eSOAP), Letterkenny University Hospital, Letterkenny, Ireland

Letterkenny University Hospital and University Hospital Galway, Letterkenny, Donegal, Ireland

© World Society of Emergency Surgery and Donegal Clinical and Research Academy 2020   155
M. Sugrue et al. (eds.), *Resources for Optimal Care of Emergency Surgery*,
Hot Topics in Acute Care Surgery and Trauma,
https://doi.org/10.1007/978-3-030-49363-9_24

24.3   Laparotomy Wound Care

A wound closure bundle to include documentation of facial closure technique, subcutaneous and skin closure techniques to ensure

Description	Documented compliance with recent advance in fascial closure and layered closure techniques
Rationale	Wound infection can be markedly reduced by a bundle approach.
Target	90% emergency abdominal surgery has compliance with ideal laparotomy closure bundle.
KPI reporting	6 monthly
Data sources	EGS registry

Complications in Emergency Surgery

25

Michael Sugrue, Kevin Blake, Brendan Skelly, and Angus J. M. Watson

25.1 Complications Tracking and Reporting System

Emergency surgery patients reported complications rate

Description	Measurement of complications
Rationale	Identifying patient-related complications. This ideally would be recorded prospectively in a computerized networked database. This system should be accessible through the hospital campus to ensure ease of entry.
Target	95% of complications occurring during hospital stay are recorded.
KPI reporting	Monthly
Data sources	EGS registry

M. Sugrue (✉)
EU INTERREG Emergency Surgery Outcomes Advancement Project (eSOAP),
Letterkenny University Hospital, Letterkenny, Donegal, Ireland

Letterkenny University Hospital and University Hospital Galway,
Letterkenny, Donegal, Ireland

K. Blake
EU Interreg, Centre for Personalised Medicine,
Letterkinny Institute of Technology, Letterkenny, Co. Donegal, Ireland
e-mail: Kevin.Blake@lyit.ie

B. Skelly
EU INTERREG Emergency Surgery Outcomes Advancement Project (eSOAP),
Letterkenny University Hospital, Letterkenny, Co. Donegal, Ireland

Department of Surgery, Altnagelvin Hospital, Derry, Northern Ireland, UK
e-mail: Brendan.Skelly@westerntrust.hscni.net

A. J. M. Watson
Department of Surgery, Raigmore Hospital, Inverness, Scotland, UK
e-mail: angus.watson@nhs.net

© World Society of Emergency Surgery and Donegal Clinical and Research Academy 2020   157
M. Sugrue et al. (eds.), *Resources for Optimal Care of Emergency Surgery*,
Hot Topics in Acute Care Surgery and Trauma,
https://doi.org/10.1007/978-3-030-49363-9_25

Complication reports have documented feedback mechanism within hospital governance

Description	Documented feedback and reporting mechanisms for complications
Rationale	The identification of complications would lead to a quality change with the hospitals clinical and organizational structure.
Target	Demonstrated quality improvement project originating from complication reporting
KPI reporting	Annually
Data sources	EGS registry

Identification of complication rates outside international norms

Description	Flagging complication rates that appear to be either superior or inferior to perceived international norms.
Rationale	This would allow sharing of systems that are associated with exceptional good results or targeting those where performance is sub-optimal.
Target	10% of reported complication rates are superior to international reported meta-analysis rates.
KPI reporting	Annually
Data sources	EGS registry

Correction to: Resources for Optimal Care of Emergency Surgery

Michael Sugrue, Ron Maier, Ernest E. Moore,
Fausto Catena, Federico Coccolini, and Yoram Kluger

Correction to:
M. Sugrue et al. (eds.), *Resources for Optimal Care of Emergency Surgery*, **Hot Topics in Acute Care Surgery and Trauma,**
https://doi.org/10.1007/978-3-030-49363-9

The original version of the book was revised: Affiliation of one of the editors, Ernest E. Moore, has been updated.

The updated online version of this book can be found at
https://doi.org/10.1007/978-3-030-49363-9

Printed in the United States
by Baker & Taylor Publisher Services